Suicide Risk Management

Suicide Risk Management

A Manual for Health Professionals 2e

Sonia Chehil
MD FRCPC
Assistant Professor of Psychiatry
Dalhousie University, Halifax, Canada

Stan Kutcher
MD FRCPC
Professor of Psychiatry
Dalhousie University, Halifax, Canada

WILEY-BLACKWELL

A John Wiley & Sons, Ltd., Publication

This edition first published 2012 © 2012 by John Wiley & Sons, Ltd.

Wiley-Blackwell is an imprint of John Wiley & Sons, formed by the merger of
Wiley's global Scientific, Technical and Medical business with Blackwell Publishing.

Registered office: John Wiley & Sons, Ltd, The Atrium, Southern Gate, Chichester, West
Sussex, PO19 8SQ, UK

Editorial offices: 9600 Garsington Road, Oxford, OX4 2DQ, UK
                       The Atrium, Southern Gate, Chichester, West Sussex, PO19 8SQ, UK
                       111 River Street, Hoboken, NJ 07030-5774, USA

For details of our global editorial offices, for customer services and for information about
how to apply for permission to reuse the copyright material
in this book please see our website at www.wiley.com/wiley-blackwell.

Library of Congress Cataloging-in-Publication Data

Kutcher, Stanley P.
   Suicide risk management : a manual for health professionals / Stan Kutcher,
Sonia Chehil. – 2nd ed.
       p. ; cm.
   Includes index.
   ISBN 978-0-470-97856-6 (pbk.)
   I. Chehil, Sonia.   II. Title.
   [DNLM: 1.   Suicide–prevention & control. 2.   Suicide–psychology. 3.   Risk
Assessment–methods. WM 165]
   LC classification not assigned
   616.85'8445–dc23

                                                                      2011030220

A catalogue record for this book is available from the British Library.

This book is published in the following electronic formats: ePDF 9781119953111; Wiley
Online Library: 9781119953128; ePub 978119954316; Mobi 9781119954323

Set in 10.5/12.5pt Times Roman by Thomson Digital, Noida, India

First Impression   2012

Contents

Introduction

Understanding suicide is unachievable. The underpinnings of suicide are diverse and multifaceted, involving a unique fusion of biological, psychosocial and cultural factors for each individual. Suicide is not an event that occurs in a vacuum. It is the ultimate consequence of a process.

For many people who take the decision to end their own life we will never be able to answer the question 'Why?' For some, self-inflicted death may be:

- an escape from despair and suffering
- a relief from intractable emotional, psychological or physical pain
- a response to a stigmatizing illness
- an escape from feelings of hopelessness
- a consequence of acute intoxication
- a response to commanding homicidal or self-harm auditory hallucinations
- a manifestation of bizarre or grandiose delusions
- a declaration of religious devotion
- a testimony of nationalist or political allegiance
- a means of atonement
- a means of reunification with a deceased loved one
- a means of rebirth
- a method of revenge
- a way to protect family honour

This does not mean that health professionals should not know how to recognize, assess and manage the suicidal patient. Indeed, all health professionals should be proficient in this core competency as many of their patients may face the prospect of suicide at some time in their lives. Many patients who experience suicidal thoughts or make suicide plans will change their minds about committing suicide. Many people who attempt suicide and are not successful go on to live productive lives. For some, a suicide attempt is an event that leads to a first contact with a helping professional. Some of these individuals may be suffering from a mental disorder that will respond to appropriate and effective treatment. Some may be suffering from chronic physical disorders; others may be overwhelmed by life stressors. In any case, many of these individuals may consider suicide as a viable solution to their problems or the only means to ending their suffering. By being aware of suicide risk factors and knowing how to identify and provide appropriate targeted interventions for suicidal individuals, health professionals can assist in the patient choosing life rather than death.

Cultural, religious, geographical and socioeconomic factors all impact on the expression of suicidality and the completion of suicide. Thus, health professionals from various countries or regions may need to adapt some of the material in this book to reflect local perspectives. However, we all need to remember, whenever a clinician and a suicidal person interact, that careful, considerate application of suicide risk management will need to be applied – regardless of context. Contexts differ but people are similar.

Objectives

1 To provide information regarding the epidemiology, risk factors and associated aspects of suicide.
2 To provide information that will assist in the understanding and assessment of suicide risk.
3 To provide a continuous self-study programme pertaining to clinical evaluation of suicide, using the Suicide Risk Assessment Guide (SRAG).
4 To introduce the Tool for Assessment of Suicide Risk (TASR) and provide instruction on its appropriate clinical application.

Chapter 1
The Importance of Suicide Awareness and Assessment

Why is it important to know about suicide?

Suicide is a significant public health problem worldwide. Suicide represents 1.4% of the Global Burden of Disease and accounts for nearly half of all violent deaths and almost one million fatalities globally each year. Although these numbers may seem alarming, it is widely believed that they are underestimates of the true global prevalence and global burden of suicide.

For every life lost to suicide there are many more left in the wake of the tragedy – parents, children, siblings, friends and communities.

'For every suicide death there are scores of family and friends whose lives are devastated emotionally, socially and economically . . . Suicide is a tragic global public health problem. Worldwide, more people die from suicide than from all homicides and wars combined. There is an urgent need for coordinated and intensified global action to prevent this needless toll.'

Dr Catherine Le Galès-Camus, WHO Assistant-Director General, World Mental Health Day 2006

Suicide Risk Management: A Manual for Health Professionals, Second Edition. Sonia Chehil and Stan Kutcher.

Challenges to understanding global suicide rates and suicide risk

Estimating suicide prevalence in different countries is problematic. Suicide rates range substantially between countries (WHO, 2009) and the variability of data collection and reporting makes national comparisons difficult if not impossible. Many countries lack a standard surveillance system that accurately captures suicide death. Where surveillance systems exist, data validity can be obscured by variability in the classification of suicide deaths, procedures for recording suicide deaths, procedures for completing death certificates, and the bodies responsible for determining the cause of unexpected death. The stigma associated with suicide is also a significant barrier to estimating true prevalence rates. In many cultures suicide is hidden by affected families to avoid shame, disgrace, ridicule or social exclusion. Worldwide, cultural, religious and social values and beliefs have significantly influenced what has been reported in official death records and are believed to continue to contribute to the misclassification of suicide deaths as accidental or due to unknown causes in many countries. Therefore, 'prevalence estimates' taken from country records globally likely underestimate actual suicide rates.

The pervasive stigma, shame and humiliation associated with a suicide death are perpetuated by legislation that continues to classify suicide as a criminal offence in many developing countries. Although such laws may now rarely, if ever, be enforced in most jurisdictions, in some, persons who survive a suicide attempt may be tried and convicted in court. So too might family members of a suicide victim be charged with stiff penalties or be subject to social humiliation. Not surprisingly, reported prevalence figures in countries where such laws are upheld are consistently reported to be extremely low. Nevertheless, based on available data, globally suicide is believed to account for an average of 10–15 deaths for every 100 000 persons each year, and for each completed suicide there are believed to be up to 20 failed suicide attempts.

Another compounding issue in understanding global and national suicide rates is the large jurisdictional variations in reported suicides even within countries where suicide data are relatively well collected. Suicide rates vary widely across different states in the USA and across provinces and territories in Canada, for example. Historically, suicide rates within jurisdictions, countries and regions have demonstrated secular trends that are poorly understood. The complexity of factors outside the suicidal individual that may contribute to increased risk is substantial. The underpinnings of suicide are diverse and multifaceted, involving a unique fusion of biological, psychosocial, political, economic and cultural factors for each individual. The significance of each factor or combination of factors in any location at any one time is difficult to deconstruct. For example, in many developed countries, including Canada and the USA, historical prevalence data demonstrate that suicide in young adults and teens started increasing in the 1950s. In the last decade and a half this longstanding trend shifted, with youth suicide rates in many developed countries decreasing or reaching a plateau. This shift has not been strongly correlated with the presence or absence of national suicide prevention strategies and it is not clear what factors have been most important in changing this suicide trend in young people, although considerations have included the more effective identification and treatment of depression and control of lethal means. Nonetheless, in the USA and many other countries (particularly in wealthy or developed states), suicide continues to be one of the three leading causes of death in young people between the ages of 15 and 24.

The majority of studies on risk factors for suicide have been conducted in developed countries using the psychological autopsy methodology. Psychological autopsy studies in the West have consistently demonstrated strong associations between suicide and mental disorder, reporting that 90% of people who die by suicide have one or more diagnosable mental illness. The most common diagnoses found to be associated with suicide death include the affective (mood) disorders, anxiety disorders, substance abuse disorders, personality disorders and schizophrenia. These studies have identified the presence of an untreated mental disorder – particularly depression and substance abuse – as the greatest attributable risk factor for suicide.

Using the same type of psychological autopsy methodology, studies conducted in developing countries have not demonstrated as robust an association between suicide and mental disorder as purported in the West. Undoubtedly there are many factors that may explain this discrepancy. In developing countries, suicide may be less clearly correlated with mental disorder and may be more often influenced by cultural, religious, social, economic and political factors. The dearth of mental health resources in most developing countries and the lack of accessible and available mental health services may lead to a systematic under-diagnosis of mental illnesses. Stigma, cultural understandings of mental health and mental disorder, and traditional methods for the care and treatment of the mentally ill may also contribute to this difference. Despite the apparent variability between studies conducted in different parts of the world, a strong and consistent association between suicide and mental disorders is undeniable. Thus, the scaling up of mental health services to improve early detection, intervention and management of mental illness – particularly in primary care, where most conditions first present – is recognized as the cornerstone of any suicide prevention strategy.

Not negating the significance of mental disorder to suicide risk, it is important to recognize that the vast majority of people with mental disorders will not die by suicide and that many people who die by suicide do not have a diagnosable mental disorder. Thus, having a mental disorder is neither necessary nor sufficient in itself to account for suicide deaths. Other identified significant risk factors include current or past suicide behaviour, availability of and access to lethal means, exposure to trauma or abuse, severe psychosocial stressors, interpersonal loss, family history of suicide and mental disorder, alcohol and drug misuse, lack of significant relationships and social isolation, chronic physical illness, disabling pain, lack of internal coping abilities, and lack of access to health and social services and supports. Thus, in addition to scaling up mental health services, suicide prevention activities must also address identified modifiable socio-cultural-political-environmental factors that influence suicide risk.

> Suicide prevention is not the purview of health alone. Suicide prevention is everyone's responsibility – individuals, families, community organizations and agencies including faith-based organizations, private business, and all levels of government – and requires a multi-sectoral response to achieve success.

Role of health professionals in suicide risk mgnt

Suicide risk assessment is a necessary core competency required by all health providers. Regardless of location or setting, health providers are often the first point of contact for individuals and families who may be at risk for suicide. In North America, studies indicate that the majority (up to two-thirds) of those who die by suicide have had contact with a health care professional for various physical and emotional complaints in the month before their death. Unfortunately, many patients who are contemplating suicide do not spontaneously voice suicidal thoughts or plans to their health care provider, and the majority of those at risk are never asked about suicidality during general clinical assessments. Consequently, individuals at risk are often never identified and do not receive needed intervention and support. Failure to identify individuals at risk for suicide may stem from a lack of training in the identification of suicide risk factors, lack of comfort or confidence on the part of the health care professional in addressing suicide risk, time and resource constraints of busy clinical practices, or a combination of these and other factors. Working with patients at risk for suicide is difficult and anxiety-provoking for many health providers. Even among mental health professionals who work with recognized populations at risk for suicide, working with a suicidal patient is considered one of the most stressful and challenging components of their clinical practice. Nonetheless, all health providers must have the knowledge, skills and competencies necessary to identify, assess and manage suicide risk with confidence, care and respect. Once the health care provider has developed necessary suicide risk-assessment competencies she/he can apply them in any setting where individual evaluation occurs.

What are some of the barriers to detection and prevention of suicide?

Several factors can impede the detection and prevention of suicide:
- stigma
- failure to seek help
- lack of suicide knowledge and awareness among health professionals
- suicide is a rare event.

Stigma

Stigma refers to the shame, disgrace or reproach attached to something that is considered socially unacceptable. In many cultures suicide is seen as shameful, sinful, weak, selfish or manipulative. These beliefs are held both by society as a whole and by those who are contemplating suicide. Stigma acts to reinforce both secrecy and silence and contributes to feelings of isolation, self-contempt and self-deprecation in individuals experiencing thoughts of suicide, and shame and guilt in those with loved ones who have committed suicide.

The social stigma of suicide is compounded by the link between mental disorder and suicide. People with mental disorders continue to be amongst the most marginalized in their society and experience greater misaddress of human rights than any other group of ill people, regardless of their religious affiliation, cultural identity or place of residence. In many parts of the world mental illness fails to be recognized as a legitimate health disorder and people with mental illness continue to be misunderstood as weak, lazy, attention seeking, crazy or stupid. Fear of being thought of or being labelled as mentally ill and fear of the ridicule, discrimination, social exclusion, loss of friends, loss of employment or loss of opportunity that may result likely contributes to the secrecy and silence that keeps people from reaching out and receiving help.

Sadly, the stigma associated with mental illness, as with suicide, is based on misinformation and misunderstanding.

Failure to seek help

As stated above, the stigma attached to suicide and the consequent fear of social sanctions, discrimination, loss of dignity and self-respect can prevent people from seeking help or disclosing suicidal thoughts and plans. For some, contemplating disclosure of suicidality may be associated with such intense feelings of personal shame, humiliation or embarrassment – as well as fear of judgment and ridicule by friends, family, community and health providers – that suffering in silence or ending their life may seem a more acceptable solution. Others may fear that disclosure will result in the forced interruption of a process to which they have committed. Some may fear loss of control over their situation or that disclosure will result in involuntary hospitalization. In jurisdictions in which suicide is considered a criminal offence, individuals may not disclose suicidal thoughts or plans for fear of

Common suicide myths that serve to support and sustain the social stigma of suicide

Myth	Reality
If someone talks about suicide they are unlikely to actually do anything to harm themselves	Many people who die by suicide have communicated their feelings, thoughts or plans before their death
Suicide is always an impulsive act	Many people who commit suicide have experienced suicidal thoughts and have contemplated taking their own life before the act
Suicide is an expected or natural response to stress	Suicide is an abnormal outcome of stress. Everybody experiences stress . . . not everybody attempts suicide
Suicide is caused by stress	Suicide attempts or acts of self-harm may sometimes occur following an acute stressor (such as the breakup of a relationship or following an intense argument) but the event is a **behavioural trigger, not a cause** of suicide
People who are **really** at risk for suicide are not ambivalent about completing the act	The intensity of suicidality waxes and wanes and many people who attempt or commit suicide struggle with their conviction to die
People who commit suicide are selfish and weak	Many people who commit suicide suffer from a mental disorder that may or may not have been recognized
Someone who is smart and successful would never commit suicide	Be careful . . . remember, suicidality is often kept secret. 'Suicide' has no cultural, ethnic, racial or socioeconomic boundaries

(continued)

Myth	Reality
Talking about suicide with a depressed person will probably cause them to commit suicide	Many depressed people who have suicidal thoughts or plans are relieved when someone knows about them and is able to help them. Discussing suicidality with a depressed person will not lead them to commit suicide
There is nothing that can be done for a person who is suicidal	Many individuals who attempt suicide may be suffering from a mental disorder that will respond to appropriate and effective treatment. Appropriate treatment of a mental disorder significantly reduces the risk of suicide. For example, suicidality associated with depression usually resolves with effective treatment of the depressive disorder
People who attempt suicide are just looking for attention	In some people a suicide attempt is an event that leads to a first contact with a helping professional. A desperate cry for help is not equivalent to wanting attention

being criminally charged and prosecuted. In cultures in which suicide is prohibited, people may fear facing public humiliation, or social and family sanction.

In some cultures self-inflicted death may be covertly sanctioned in specific sociocultural contexts, for example suicides committed in the name of family honour. In these circumstances, silence, shame and secrecy may be attributed to both the act itself and the circumstances preceding the act. In other situations, religious or secular authorities may overtly sanction suicide that is committed as an act of martyrdom. In these cases, public expression of self-inflicted death may be seen as a declaration of religious devotion, nationalism or political belief.

Regardless of the reasons, many of those who die by suicide do not seek help and do not inform others of their plans. Moreover, some who are contemplating suicide or who are committed to completing suicide may not reveal their thoughts or plans even when directly asked. Thus, asking about suicidal ideation or plan does not ensure that accurate or complete information will be received or that suicide will always be prevented. This, however, does not mean that health professionals should not conduct appropriate suicide assessments when known risk factors are present. Indeed, empathic questioning of high-risk individuals about suicidal thoughts, intents or plans from a knowledgeable and caring health professional will often be seen as an expression of support, interest and professional competency. Such questioning can often encourage the suicidal individual to seek help.

Lack of suicide knowledge and awareness among health professionals

Suicide assessment and intervention are often not components of health professional school training programmes, nor are they a component of most routine general health assessment and evaluation procedures and protocols. Consequently, many health providers do not have the opportunity to develop the skills necessary to feel competent to ask about suicidality or to manage suicidal patients. Further, health providers are not immune to the cultural idioms and stigma associated with suicide.

A common misconception among health professionals is that talking to patients about suicide will increase the likelihood of the patient engaging in suicidal behaviours or dying by suicide. This is not the case. Asking a patient about suicidal thoughts will not plant or nurture these thoughts in the patient's mind. Rather, patients with suicidal thoughts often feel relieved that they have been given 'permission' to talk about them. Many patients who have suicidal ideation feel burdened, ashamed and/or sinful for having such thoughts. Some are frightened by these thoughts. Some interpret these thoughts as reinforcements for their own perceived worthlessness. Opening a dialogue about suicidality in a nonjudgmental and respectful manner can provide the patient with the opportunity to break their silence, discuss their circumstances, express their thoughts and feelings, and decompress their psychological and emotional pain. In fact, for those patients for whom suicide has become their 'only perceived option', disclosure may provide the opportunity to explore alternative choices that they have been unable to see.

Talking about suicide with a caring and nonjudgemental health provider can help a person choose life rather than choosing death.

Suicide is a rare event

Another issue that interferes with the prevention of completed suicide is the relative rarity of the event itself. As mentioned above, suicide attempts occur much more frequently than completed suicides (up to 20 times more frequently!) and suicidal ideation (having thoughts of wanting to die or of killing oneself) is more common still (up to 6 times more common than suicide attempts and up to 100 times more common than completed suicides!). Hence, most people who have suicidal thoughts and many of those who make a suicide attempt never die from suicide.

Because suicide is a rare event, it is not considered useful to screen entire populations for suicide thoughts or to routinely ask every single patient about suicidal ideas at every health professional contact. A number of risk factors, however, have been identified that can provide clinicians with a risk profile for suicide. Health professionals who are familiar with these risk factors can thereby identify potential 'at-risk' patients for assessment of suicide risk.

Can we always predict who will or who will not die by suicide?

Unfortunately, the answer is 'no'. What we can do is assess individual 'suicide risk' based on identified suicide risk and suicide protective factors that may help identify those who are more or less likely to attempt or complete suicide in the near future. The health professional approaches the issue of suicide in the clinical setting by estimating the burden of risk at a point in time. *How strong is the risk for suicide in the near future*? This is determined by learning how to identify and weigh both risk and protective factors. A clinical decision is then formulated as to whether suicide risk is high, moderate or low.

Suicide risk evaluation is not an exact science. Each individual's composite 'risk' is estimated based on the presence, relevance and weighting of risk and protective factors for that individual, taking into consideration their psychosocial and cultural context and their life experience at the time of assessment. The relevance and weighting of risk and protective factors are not universal and certain risk factors when present simultaneously may increase risk exponentially in one context but not in another.

While it may be possible to be relatively certain in one's risk prediction for the near future, it is almost impossible to be certain in one's risk prediction outside a window of three to seven days, or thereabouts. That is why for individuals who demonstrate some degree of risk, evaluation of risk potential becomes an ongoing process. Changes in the psychosocial, occupational, health or mental health status of a person at low risk may move that individual into a higher-risk category.

While it is not possible to always predict who will or will not die by suicide, being aware of warning signs for suicide risk and being comfortable and competent in the application of an appropriate suicide risk assessment can assist the health provider in the early detection, assessment and management of patients at risk of suicide and the implementation of appropriate immediate, short-term and ongoing interventions that can assist an individual in choosing life rather than death.

Important definitions

Suicidality   Any thoughts or actions associated with an implicit or explicit intent to die. This includes suicide ideation, suicide intent, suicide plans and suicide attempts.

Suicidal ideation   Thoughts, images or fantasies of harming or killing oneself.

Suicide attempt   A purposeful self-inflicted act that is nonfatal and is associated with implicit or explicit intent to die.

Completed suicide   A purposeful self-inflicted act that is fatal and is associated with implicit or explicit intent to die

Self-harm (or self-injurious behaviour)   Purposeful self-inflicted acts that are not associated with an implicit or explicit intent to die. The intent of self-harm is often to reduce distress and it is used as a coping strategy, albeit an unhealthy strategy, to manage distressing thoughts and feelings.

Suicide behaviours   Any purposeful self-inflicted acts, including suicide attempts, self-harm and self-injury, that may lead to death, regardless of the intent of those behaviours and actions.

Chapter 2
Understanding Suicide Risk

Suicide: protective factors and risk factors

A myriad of risk factors have been associated with suicide death in both developing and developed countries. Although there do appear to be some universal risk factors, such as the presence of a mental disorder, youth or old age, low socioeconomic status, substance abuse, previous suicide attempts and recent stressful life events, there are also notable differences. Even amongst the universal risk factors, the significance and weighting of each is not necessarily universal across nations. In addition, there are notable cultural, regional and country-specific differences. This chapter will present a selective review of factors associated with suicide death, reflecting largely data from developed countries.

Suicide and suicide behaviours are influenced by risk and protective factors across a person's lifespan. Risk factors and protective factors may be distal or proximal, modifiable or nonmodifiable, and work together to influence a person's suicide risk. Suicide prevention strategies target modifiable risk and protective factors, striving to reduce risk factors and increase protective factors at individual, community and population levels. Identification of factors that may increase or decrease a patient's level of suicide risk can help clinicians to establish an estimate of the overall level of suicide risk for an individual patient, and this in turn can assist in the development of

Suicide Risk Management: A Manual for Health Professionals, Second Edition.
Sonia Chehil and Stan Kutcher.
© 2012 John Wiley & Sons, Ltd. Published 2012 by John Wiley & Sons, Ltd.

treatment plans that best address patient safety and target identified modifiable physical, behavioural, psychosocial, environmental and personality factors.

It is important to remember, however, that **no one protective or risk factor** independently in and of itself can determine the event of suicide. Also, not all protective or risk factors are equally strong in prediction. For example, whereas gender is a risk factor (males are more likely to commit suicide than females in most countries studied), having a suicidal plan poses a much greater degree of risk than being male. When thinking about protective and risk factors for suicide it is important to think about these factors in aggregate and to view them within the context of the patient's experience. This will help you weigh how strong the risk will be for each individual patient.

Protective factors for suicide

Protective factors are those factors and experiences that are believed to reduce the risk for suicide and suicide behaviours and increase a person's ability to cope with and manage stress and face life's challenges. Protective factors can be divided into 'internal' and 'external' factors. For individuals presenting with suicidality or a suicide attempt, the ability to identify 'reasons for living' is considered an important 'internal' protective factor against suicide. For one, it argues against 'hopelessness' and 'pessimism' by focusing individuals on what they have in their lives and promoting feelings of optimism. Connection to others, guilt about hurting loved ones, religious beliefs, pregnancy, children and a sense of responsibility to family are some of the protective 'reasons for living' cited by individuals with suicidal ideation. Other internal protective factors include strong coping and problem-solving skills; interpersonal competence; high life satisfaction; strong sense of belonging and connection to self, family and community; sense of purpose; being future-focused; experience with success, mastery and self-effectiveness; confidence in being able to overcome adversity; strong cultural identity; and strong connection to faith. Examples of external protective factors include having a strong network of support and acceptance; having supports that are available and accessible; healthy interpersonal relationships; cohesive community; being gainfully employed; having a good work environment; and the presence of young children in the home.

Protective factors are less well established than are risk factors and the scientific data to support their notation is generally not very strong. Regardless, the importance of understanding the role of protective factors in potentially mitigating risk for suicide and suicide behaviour, in informing the development of programmes to address suicide prevention, and in the development of individual strength-based interventions, cannot be overstated.

Factors that are thought to protect the patient against suicide include the following

- having reasons for living
- internal strengths:
  o positive self-esteem and self-efficacy
  o effective interpersonal skills
  o effective problem-solving skills
  o adaptive coping
  o intact reality-testing
  o good frustration and distress tolerance
  o strong sense of purpose or meaning
  o high life satisfaction
  o religious affiliation
  o sense of responsibility to family
  o optimism and future-focus
  o good physical and mental health
- external strengths:
  o positive social support
  o healthy personal relationships
  o strong community cohesiveness
  o employment
  o children in the home.

In the opinion of the authors of this manual, these factors have not been adequately demonstrated to prevent suicide. Many of them are simply negative restatements of known risk factors (such as absence of a mental disorder, intact reality-testing, high life satisfaction, unemployment, etc.). Thus, during an assessment of suicide risk in an individual, they should not be used to override those factors that identify suicide risk.

Risk factors for suicide

A number of risk factors have been strongly linked to both suicide and suicide behaviours. Distal risk factors can be understood as predisposing factors that may increase a person's vulnerability to suicide. Identified distal risk factors for suicide include biological factors (genetic vulnerability, neurobiology, family history of psychiatric disorder, family history of suicide and family history of violence and abuse), individual factors (history of mental disorder, previous suicide behaviours, 'exposure' to suicide – through direct or indirect personal experience, media, culture), personality characteristics (rigid cognitive style, poor coping skills, impulsivity, aggression, hypersensitivity/anxiety), early negative environmental factors (isolation, impoverished environment, lack of healthy attachments) and early traumatic life experience (loss of a parent or caregiver, trauma, neglect, and emotional, physical and sexual abuse).

Proximal risk factors include factors which augment current vulnerability for suicide as well as factors which may precipitate or trigger suicide or suicide behaviours. Proximal risk factors include recent or current suicidality and suicide behaviours; unstable and unhealthy interpersonal relationships; lack of access to health and support services; the presence of a psychiatric or significant medical condition; alcohol and substance misuse; intoxication; experience of domestic violence or abuse; access and availability of lethal means; recent loss or bereavement; recent exposure to suicide; poor cognitive and social skills; poor social supports or social isolation; recent experience of failure, shame, humiliation, rejection, loss or trauma; and current, evolving or anticipated psychosocial crisis.

Risk factors for suicide will be considered under ten headings, noted below. The presence of one or more of these risk factors may increase an individual's risk for suicide but does not necessarily predict suicide. The recognition of risk factors can assist the health professional in identifying who may require a comprehensive assessment and in formulating the overall level of an individual's risk for suicide. As previously stated, not all risk factors carry the same predictive weight and combinations of factors may increase risk exponentially or additively. It is the number, duration, severity and relative weight of each factor applied to an individual at the time of assessment and within the context of their life story that can help establish the degree of risk for suicide in the near future.

The headings are:

1 Age
2 Gender
3 Current suicidality
4 Past suicidality and suicide behaviours
5 Psychiatric history
6 Psychiatric symptoms
7 Medical history
8 Family history
9 Personal history
10 Personality

Age

In North America, Western Europe (including the UK) and most other countries for which data are available, suicide rates generally increase with increasing age. Projected on top of this trend are three peaks representing periods of increased risk: adolescence/young adulthood, middle age and old age. In general, suicide rates rise sharply in late adolescence and early adulthood, before leveling off through early midlife, then rising again in middle age and then again after age 70.

In developed countries the highest suicide rates are found in the elderly. The significance of suicide in the elderly is often underappreciated and is overshadowed by the proportionally higher contribution of other causes of mortality (including health-related causes) to 'all deaths' in this age group. In general, suicide behaviours in the elderly are more likely to be lethal as compared to younger age groups. Elders who commit suicide tend to be more socially isolated, rigid in their thinking, and generally demonstrate a greater determination to die than younger individuals, as evidenced by the fact that suicidal elders give fewer warning signs of their ideas and plans, use more violent and potentially lethal methods to commit suicide, and engage in suicidal behaviours that involve greater planning and resolve. Case fatality in elders may also be higher due to the fact that the elderly are generally less physically resilient, are more likely to be suffering from a variety of physical illnesses and are more likely to have access to medication which taken in excess or in combination have a high likelihood of lethality.

Among the 15–24-year-old age group, suicide rates in the USA tripled in the decades following the 1950s and became the third leading cause of death in young people. Over the past decade youth suicide has actually been decreasing in the USA, Canada and many (but not all) other countries. Nonetheless, in many of these countries, suicide continues to be one of the three leading causes of death in young people between the ages of 15 and 24 years. In contextualizing the contribution of suicide deaths to 'all deaths' in youth it is important to recognize that death due to other causes (apart from accidents and homicide) is proportionately lower in this age group, and contrary to popular opinion, the highest suicide rates in the first three decades of life are not in teenagers but in adults.

Question

What accounts for the rise in suicide rates during adolescence and young adulthood?

Answer

There is no simple answer to this question. A complex interplay of psychosocial and biological factors in the context of emotional, cognitive, physical and behavioural development is likely involved. The rise in suicide rates in youth, however, is strongly correlated with the rise in the incidence of mental illness. Many of the major mental disorders have their onset in adolescence. As severe mental disorders (depression, bipolar disorder, schizophrenia) increase, so do suicide rates. Contrary to much popular opinion, suicide is not caused by the usual and expected stresses of adolescence! The vast majority of young people negotiate through their teens successfully.

Gender

Suicide rates increase with increasing age in both men and woman and follow a similar general pattern across different age groups. In most countries, suicide deaths occur more frequently in men than in women. In the United States, suicide rates are four times higher in men. This disproportionate number of male deaths may be partially explained by the propensity of men to choose methods of committing suicide – such as shooting or hanging – that leave little chance for rescue and survival. Women more often choose less lethal methods, such as overdose, that allow more opportunity for rescue.

Factors that may contribute to higher suicide rates in men compared with women

- Men are less likely to seek help for emotional or psychological problems than women.
- Men may be more behaviourally impulsive than women.
- Men tend to be less socially connected than women.
- Men may be less willing to accept help for emotional or psychological problems than women.
- Men may choose more lethal suicide methods than women.
- Men may allow less chance of interruption and rescue.
- Men may have higher rates of substance abuse.
- Alcohol and substance abuse more often accompany depression in men than in women.

Question

Are there risk factors unique to women?

Answer

Female suicide behaviour, suicide attempts and completed suicide are highly correlated with domestic violence and abuse. Domestic violence and abuse can happen to anyone, irrespective of age, gender, vocation, status, culture, religion or geography, but woman are the most common victims. A woman's abuser is most often a member of her own family or her intimate partner. Globally an estimated one in three woman have experienced physical, sexual or emotional abuse in their lifetime, yet domestic violence and abuse is often undetected, overlooked, ignored, excused, denied or kept hidden in homes and communities around the world. Psychological or emotional abuse, which leaves no visible evidence but can leave deep and long lasting scars, is often minimized or not even considered to be 'abuse'.

In some cultures the gender inequalities that women face, not only in civil society but also within the family, may increase their risk for suicide. Sociocultural and familial definitions and expectations of the female 'role' or position in family and society may also be a risk factor in individual cases. The value placed on female virtue and family honour must not be underestimated, particularly in societies or groups in which these ideals are strongly embedded. In such cases, actual or perceived transgression against these values can lead to social, spousal or family sanctions that are powerful enough to compel suicidal behaviour.

Although pregnancy has been reported to be a protective factor against suicide in women, unplanned or unwanted pregnancy – which may bring severe shame, humiliation or retribution to the woman or the woman's family – is an exception. In addition, severe psychiatric illness following delivery (postpartum depression or postpartum psychosis) is associated with a higher risk of suicide as well as infanticide in women.

Postpartum depression

Fifty per cent of women will experience intense emotional symptoms including depressed mood, irritability, mood swings, crying spells, fatigue and anxiety following the delivery of a child. These symptoms usually occur within the first two weeks after giving birth and are referred to as the 'postpartum blues'.

The postpartum blues are self-limiting, usually lasting several days, rarely more than a few weeks, and do not require medical intervention apart from reassurance and monitoring. The postpartum blues, however, may be a harbinger for a more serious problem, postpartum depression (PPD).

PPD affects 10–15% of women and usually develops within the first 4–6 weeks after childbirth. Women who experience PPD meet full criteria for a major depressive episode but tend to experience more mood fluctuation and more prominent anxiety symptoms compared with a non-postpartum-related depressive episode.

Some mothers with PPD demonstrate frank disinterest in the newborn or may become fearful of being left alone with the baby. Others may become inappropriately preoccupied with the baby's wellbeing. This preoccupation may become obsessional and in some cases may reach delusional proportions. Mothers with PPD often experience feelings of intense shame, guilt and incompetence in their role as care provider for their newborn, feelings that are often inadvertently reinforced by family, community and health care providers who do not recognize the presence of an underlying disorder. Perinatal and postnatal support providers (i.e. physicians, nurses, midwives), community workers, and primary and paediatric care providers must be aware of the signs, symptoms and risk factors for PPD, and mothers experiencing symptoms of PPD must be evaluated. As with depression itself, PPD is associated with an increased risk of suicide, and may be associated with neglect of the newborn and in severe cases (particularly when associated with psychosis) infanticide.

Postpartum psychosis

Postpartum psychosis (PPP) is estimated to occur in 1 in 1000 childbirths. This disorder is believed to be closely associated with the mood disorders (bipolar and major depressive disorder). Approximately 50% of women who experience PPP have a family history of mood disorder.

Some 50–60% of women affected are primiparous (first delivery) and many (50%) have a history of perinatal (delivery) complications.

The first symptoms of PPP usually begin within the first 2 weeks following delivery. Many of the initial symptoms of PPP may be reminiscent of the postpartum blues: depressed mood, irritability, mood swings, crying spells, fatigue and anxiety. In the early stages of the illness, before the onset of frank psychosis, these symptoms are often accompanied by agitation and insomnia. Later, symptoms such as suspiciousness, cognitive deficits (confusion and incoherence) and obsessive concern about the baby's health and welfare may develop. Many women with PPP develop delusional beliefs involving the child: beliefs that the child is possessed or evil, that the child is dead, or that the child is defective. Some mothers may deny the pregnancy and birth, fear or loathe the child, or have impulses to harm the child. Persecutory and somatic delusions are also common. In addition, women with PPP may develop hallucinations, which may include command-type auditory hallucinations telling them to harm themselves and/or the baby and other children in the home. Approximately 5% of mothers affected by PPP are believed to commit suicide and up to 4% commit infanticide.

Question

Are the age and gender demographics different in developing countries?

Answer

The demographics of suicide and suicide victims in Eastern countries are quite different from those seen in the West. Although the general trend across the lifespan is similar to that seen in the West, in many Eastern nations a larger proportion of young people and women commit suicide than in the West, and the second peak in later life is less striking. There is also greater variability in the ratio of male to female suicide deaths across developing nations as compared to developed countries. Some countries, such as Pakistan, report two to three male suicides for every female death. In other countries this gender ratio is much lower. In many Asian countries, including India for example, the rates of suicide death, particularly in rural areas, are almost equal for men and women. In China, female suicide rates are 25% higher than male suicide rates.

Summary of risk factors associated with age and gender

	Higher risk	Lower risk
Age	Elderly 15–35 years	Prepubertal
Gender	Male	Female
Women	Intimate partner abuse	Pregnancy
	Domestic violence and abuse	Young children in the home
	Postpartum depression (PPD)	Strong sense of responsibility to family
	Postpartum psychosis (PPP)	
	Rigid role expectations	
	Institutionalized gender inequality	

Current suicidality

Suicidality includes any thoughts or actions associated with an implicit or explicit intent to end one's life or die by suicide. Suicidality includes suicide ideation, suicide intent, suicide plans and suicide attempts.

Suicide ideation is not uncommon. Many people may think about suicide during times of stress or crisis but the vast majority of people who have had such thoughts will never attempt or complete suicide. Nonetheless, the presence of suicidal ideation is a strong indicator of increased risk for suicide.

Thoughts of suicide can arise as an attempt by an individual to search for solutions to a problem for which there appear to be few viable options. For a person who is unable to see, or believes they have exhausted, alternative solutions, 'suicide' can become a plausible option. Thoughts of suicide can initiate the 'suicide process', which can ultimately lead to suicide action and suicide death. The suicidal process is the timespan between suicidal ideation and suicide action. Understanding the nature of the suicidal process, its duration, and the modifiable factors influencing its progression, is essential for planning successful interventions aimed at interrupting this process and preventing the act of suicide.

Suicidal ideation

Suicidal ideation refers to thoughts, fantasies, ruminations and pre-occupations about death, self-harm and self-inflicted death.

Suicidal ideation can be both 'passive' and 'active'. A person who is actively thinking about killing themselves and is having thoughts of initiating a suicide process that will lead to their death is experiencing **active suicide ideation**. A person who has thoughts about wanting to 'disappear', wishing they could just go to sleep and never wake up, or thoughts that they would rather not be alive, but who does not have thoughts of actively initiating a suicide process that would lead to their death, is experiencing **passive suicide ideation**.

Active suicide ideation confers greater risk than passive suicide ideation and the greater the magnitude and persistence of the suicidal thoughts, the higher the risk for eventual suicide.

Recall from the last chapter that many people who are contemplating suicide do not disclose their thoughts or plans before acting to end their lives. Keeping suicidality hidden or 'secret' is not uncommon. Suicidality that is not openly disclosed or is kept hidden is referred to as **'concealed' suicidality**. Concealed suicidality may confer greater risk of suicide death because the opportunity for intervention may never be identified.

Suicide ideation occurs along a continuum of frequency (fleeting to persistent), intensity (manageable to intolerable or uncontrollable), duration (chronic to acute) and persistence (intermittent to persistent), and can be associated with different levels of intent (no wish or desire to die to strong desire to die) as well as motivation.

> The presence and nature of suicide thoughts, the presence of a suicide plan, and the intent and commitment to follow through with suicide plans strongly impact the estimation of an individual's imminent risk for suicide.

Suicidal intent

Suicidal intent refers to a patient's desire and commitment to die by suicide. The level of intent can be estimated from the patient's commitment to and expectation of a chosen method or plan. The stronger the patient's commitment to carrying out a plan and the greater the expectation and belief that the plan will be lethal, the greater the risk for suicide.

Suicidal plan

The more detailed and specific the suicide plan, the greater the level of suicide risk. Risk is influenced by the lethality of the chosen method of harm, the chosen timing and setting of the event, the accessibility of the method chosen, and actions taken by the patient to prepare for the event. In general, suicide plans that are premeditated and well thought out (writing a suicide note, preparing a will, giving away personal belongings or property, securing or ensuring access to means or method of suicide), involve a highly lethal method (firearm or hanging) and involve a setting and time at which discovery is unlikely are indicative of high risk for suicide.

The suicide method chosen is a significant factor in determining risk of death by suicide. The higher the lethality of the chosen method, the higher the likelihood of suicide death. Access to and availability of specific means for suicide as well as traditional sociocultural patterns in the methods used for suicide strongly affect the prevalence of suicide methods of choice across jurisdictions. In general, men tend to choose more violent means and women less violent means. Globally, hanging, firearms and poisoning are the most common lethal means for suicide – hanging being the most common in both genders.

Firearms are the most common method of suicide in the United States. In Canada, hanging is the most common method. In developing countries, particularly in agricultural areas, ingestion of pesticides is the most common method of suicide. Although pesticide suicides are rare in Canada, the United States and most of Europe, an estimated 30% of suicide deaths globally are attributable to the ingestion of pesticide.

Question

Are there specific aspects of a suicide plan that may be associated with higher lethality?

Answer

Important aspects of a suicide plan that are suggestive of the plan's potential lethality include: the chosen method, the availability of means, the individual's understanding and belief about the lethality of the chosen method, the chance of rescue, the steps taken to enact the plan, and the individual's preparedness for death.

- **Chosen method** The choice of a higher-lethality method is associated with higher suicide risk. High-lethality methods include hanging, use of a firearm, jumping from heights, pesticide ingestion and motor vehicle accidents.
- **Availability of means** The easier it is for the patient to access lethal means, the higher the risk.
- **Expected outcome** The patient's belief in the lethality of the method reflects the patient's intent and commitment to die.
- **Chance of rescue** A lower chance of rescue is associated with higher risk of successful suicide.
- **Steps taken to enact the plan** Actions taken to carry out the plan, such as purchasing a firearm, hoarding pills, establishing the date, time and setting for the event, and ensuring isolation and low risk of discovery, all increase suicide risk.
- **Preparedness for death** Plans made by patients to set their affairs in order may be indicative of anticipated death by suicide (i.e. plans made to meet financial obligations, making of a will, discarding possessions, writing letters to loved ones, making amends with others, and formulating a suicide note).

Summary of current suicidality risk factors

	Higher risk	Lower risk
Suicide ideation	Persistent Intense Uncontrollable Acute Prolonged	Fleeting Low-intensity Manageable
Suicide intent	Strong desire to die Strong commitment to act Expectation of death	High ambivalence Low commitment to act
Suicide plans	Premeditated Well planned Highly lethal means Access to means	No plan Low lethality Method No access to means

Past suicidality and suicide behaviours

Self-harm refers to deliberate self-injurious behaviours that are not associated with an implicit or explicit intent to die. Common self-harm behaviours include cutting, burning, hitting, ingestion of toxic substances and asphyxiation. The lack of intent to die or end one's life distinguishes self-harm from a suicide attempt. The 'intent' of self-harm behaviours may include the release of tension, anxiety or pressure; reduction of emotional or psychological pain; self-punishment; controlling or avoiding negative thoughts and feelings; help-seeking; or manipulation. A common misconception regarding self-harm behaviour is that because the intent is not to die people who self-harm are not at risk of suicide. This is untrue. Self-harm behaviour may be a symptom of an underlying mental disorder, serious mental health problems, and/or acute (or acute on chronic) psychosocial stress. Although the intention of self-harm may not be to end one's life, people who self-harm are at increased risk of accidental death as well as suicide.

Suicide attempts are 10–20 times more prevalent than completed suicides and up to 50% of those who die by suicide have made at least one previous attempt. These figures are likely underestimates of the true prevalence of suicide attempts as many attempts likely go undetected unless they are severe enough to warrant medical attention. In addition, most planned attempts that are in evolution but are aborted are unlikely ever to be captured. Although most individuals who make a suicide attempt do not attempt again and will not die by suicide, past suicide attempts are a major risk factor for suicide death. Up to one-fifth of people who attempt suicide will reattempt (most within a year) and reattempts are often associated with more lethal means, lower chance of rescue and survival, and higher likelihood of serious medical consequences.

History of a past suicide attempt is the best predictor of future suicide

Self-harm behaviours and suicide attempts are more common in younger age groups than in the elderly and are more common in woman than men. The higher rates of suicide attempts in woman may reflect gender differences in choice of means for suicide – men tending to choose more lethal and violent means that make survival less likely as compared to woman. In some jurisdictions self-harm behaviours are reported as 'suicide attempts' and in such cases the gender differences in suicide attempts may be erroneously inflated.

For individuals who have attempted suicide in the past, the risk of completed suicide is increased if the past attempt was recent, if there is a history of multiple past attempts, if the patient regrets having survived a past attempt, or if past attempts were associated with strong intent to die, involved methods of high lethality, led to serious adverse consequences (such as medical complications) or were premeditated with measures taken to avoid discovery. In addition, the presence of a longstanding medical illness or psychiatric condition (particularly depression or alcohol abuse), social isolation and poor social supports increases the risk of future suicide death in people who have attempted suicide.

Characteristics of past attempts that increase future suicide risk

- recency
- high number
- high intent to die
- regret over failure/survival
- use of highly lethal means
- resulting adverse consequences
- premeditation and good planning
- low chance of discovery.

Individuals factors that increase risk of future attempts and death by suicide

- presence of a longstanding medical illness
- presence of psychiatric illness
- social isolation
- lack of social supports.

Summary of past suicide behaviour risk factors

Past suicidal behaviours associated with increased suicide risk	Higher risk	Lower risk
Detected suicide attempts	Recent attempt	First attempt
Undetected suicide attempts	Multiple past attempts	Grateful for survival
Aborted suicide attempts	High intent to die	Regret of attempt
Self-harm and self-injurious behaviours	Regret of survival	High ambivalence
	Use of highly lethal means	Low intent
	Serious adverse consequences	Low-lethality method
	Premeditated and well planned	High chance of rescue
	Low chance of discovery	

Psychiatric history

Psychiatric disorder is the strongest attributable risk factor for suicide. Psychiatric disorders with the highest associated risk include the mood disorders, substance abuse (particularly alcohol) disorders, anxiety disorders, psychotic disorders and personality disorders. In addition, the presence of depressive symptoms, hopelessness or comorbid alcohol- or other substance-use disorders increases risk when found concurrently with any psychiatric disorder.

Before beginning a discussion of the risk factors associated with the different disorders, let's review the relationship between suicide and mental disorders.

Understanding suicide and mental disorder

The risk and protective factors for suicide significantly overlap with the risk and protective factors associated with the development of, or poor outcomes related to, mental disorder. Genetic vulnerability, family history, early negative life experiences such as child abuse and neglect, early environmental insults (perinatal complications), impoverished environment, low socioeconomic status, trauma exposure, and significant negative life events are associated with both suicidality and risk for mental health problems and mental disorders. In addition, the symptoms of mental disorders may be directly involved with the development of suicidal behaviours. Command hallucinations in patients experiencing psychosis is one example. The hopelessness, worthlessness, and social and emotional isolation characterizing major depressive disorder is another.

Mental disorders are characterized by disturbances in emotion, thinking and behaviour. Mental illness can diminish one's capacity for rational thought, problem-solving, judgment, impulse control and self-regulation (a person's ability to regulate their internal and external emotional responses and behaviours). Mental illness can interfere with a person's volition, motivation and ability to meaningfully engage in social, vocational and recreational activities. In addition, people living with mental disorder are more likely than the general population to suffer discrimination, abuse and social exclusion; be unmarried; lack strong social supports; fail to meet internal and external goals for personal, social and vocational achievement; and fail to fulfil social, cultural and familial roles and expectations. People with mental disorders are also more likely to drop out of school and to be unemployed and unskilled. People with mental disorders are thus less likely to have many of the important protective factors that may mitigate suicide risk, including the coping and problem-solving skills, cognitive capacity and general resilience to manage negative life events and crisis situations. Individuals suffering from a mental illness who are socially isolated; who have experienced significant personal, academic, vocational or financial loss; who have maladaptive coping skills; who have, as a consequence of their illness, become dependent on others; who have lost previously held skills or social status; or who are no longer able to fulfil their sociocultural-familial role may be at particularly high risk for suicide.

Factors that may increase suicide risk in individuals with any psychiatric disorder:
- social isolation
- loss of family role/status
- interpersonal losses
- vocational/occupational loss

- loss of previous skills/competencies
- awareness of deficits with recovery
- substance or alcohol abuse/dependence
- poor problem-solving capacity (cognitive impairment)
- depressive symptoms
- hopelessness.

Mood disorders

Mood disorders confer a 20-fold increased risk of death by suicide. It is estimated that 50% of people who die by suicide may suffer from a **major depressive disorder**. Major depressive disorder and the depressive and mixed phases of bipolar disorder are the diagnoses most often associated with suicide deaths. Individuals experiencing a depressive episode within the context of a bipolar illness may be at higher risk for suicide than those who experience a depressive episode within the context of a unipolar illness (major depressive disorder). Clinical depression affects 6–8% of the population. First onset is often in adolescence or early adulthood and is highly co-related with the increased suicide rates among youth. It is a chronic episodic illness, with the great majority of individuals experiencing a further episode within five years of the onset of the first. Although recent research has demonstrated genetic propensities to depression, suicidal behaviour in depression is the output of a complex interplay between illness and environmental factors.

For younger patients suffering from major depressive disorder or bipolar disorder, suicides are more likely to occur early in the illness course, particularly if depressive symptoms are accompanied by panic attacks, severe anxiety, diminished concentration, severe insomnia, alcohol abuse or anhedonia (loss of pleasure or interest in previously enjoyed activities). The presence of hopelessness, ranging from pessimism and negative expectation about the future to despairing about the future, has also been associated with increased suicide risk, particularly in later stages of the illness. When depression occurs concurrently with a chronic medical condition (such as pain or heart disease) or a life-threatening medical disorder (such as cancer) suicide risk may be substantially increased.

By convention, clinical depression is diagnosed following syndromal criteria spelled out in one of two diagnostic classification systems: the DSM or the ICD (International Classification of Disease). In general, individuals must demonstrate most of the following symptoms, and the symptoms must be different than their usual mood state, have persisted over time and have led to functional impairment:
- depressed, sad or irritable mood
- loss of interest or pleasure
- lack of energy
- difficulty in concentration
- loss of appetite
- thoughts and feelings of worthlessness or hopelessness
- guilty ruminations
- pronounced sleep difficulties
- suicidal ideation/plans (or the feeling that life is not worth living).

Although some patients with depression will present with emotional or psychological complaints, many may present with one or more persistent physical symptom such as difficulty sleeping, weakness, headaches, lack of energy, digestive problems and other vague or nonspecific complaints for which there is no clear medical cause. In other cases, patients, or their family members, may present with concerns about a sudden or gradual decline in physical, work, school, social or family functioning. In these clinical scenarios, further enquiry may reveal underlying core depressive symptoms such as low mood, loss of interest or irritability. Thus, health professionals must be alert to a range of presenting problems that may be 'warning signs' accompanying or concealing depression.

Every depressed patient should have ongoing monitoring of suicide risk – even when they are 'feeling better' or 'getting well'. This is particularly important during the period early in treatment as initial improvements in energy or the behavioural side effects of some medications may increase risk of suicidal thoughts or self-harm behaviours.

In addition to the diagnosis itself, the presence of specific symptoms occurring within the depressive syndrome may be associated with increased suicide risk. These include:
- hopelessness
- panic attacks

- severe anxiety
- severe anhedonia
- psychosis

High levels of hopelessness alone, with or without a diagnosis of depression, have been associated with an increased likelihood of suicidal behaviours.

Alcohol- and substance-use disorders

Alcohol abuse or dependence may play a role in 25–50% of deaths by suicide and is associated with a sixfold increased suicide mortality rate compared with the general population and a lifetime risk for suicide of up to 15%. Suicide rates are even higher among alcoholics with comorbid clinical depression. Major depressive episodes can be identified in up to three-quarters of alcoholics who die by suicide. The co-existence of a mental disorder – particularly a mood disorder, personality disorder, anxiety disorder or schizophrenia – with an alcohol- or other substance-use disorder significantly increases the risk of suicide and suicide behaviours beyond that attributable to either the mental disorder or substance-use disorder alone. Substance abuse, including polysubstance abuse, may also be a common precursor to suicide. In contrast to depression and schizophrenia, suicide among substance abusers often occurs late in the disease course, after the chronic effects of the disorder have heavily impacted on health, social, interpersonal, economic and vocational/occupational functioning. In addition to being at higher risk for completed suicide, patients with substance-use disorders, particularly alcohol abuse or dependence, are at high risk for self-inflicted harm and suicide attempts. Risk for suicide among patients with alcohol-use disorders is increased in both males and females, but as with suicide generally, the rate of completed suicide is higher in men and the rate of suicide attempts is greater in women.

Substance-use disorders: additional risk factors for suicide

- recent, impending or threatened loss or disruption of a close interpersonal relationship
- presence of other psychiatric disorders particularly depression

Alcohol-use disorders: additional risk factors for suicide
- communications of suicidal intent
- previous suicide attempts
- continued or heavier drinking
- psychosocial stressors or crisis such as loss of employmnet, legal difficulties, financial difficulties
- living alone
- poor social support
- serious medical illness
- personality disturbance
- other substance use.

Question

Can alcohol intoxication itself be a risk factor for suicide even if the person does not have alcohol abuse or dependence?

Answer

Alcohol intoxication itself, even in the absence of alcohol abuse or dependence, may be a risk factor for suicide. A significant proportion of those who die by suicide are found to have ingested alcohol before their attempt. Those who consume alcohol before committing suicide may be more likely to be experiencing an interpersonal or other psychosocial stressor and less likely to have sought help before death. Suicide in the context of alcohol intoxication may be more likely to be impulsive rather than planned and may be more likely to involve a highly lethal method such as a firearm.

Anxiety disorders

Suicidal ideation and suicide attempts are common in individuals with anxiety disorders. Anxiety disorders may play a role in 15–20% of suicides and confer a 6–10% increase in suicide risk, particularly if associated with panic attacks, depression and/or alcohol use. The presence of severe anxiety or panic attacks, within or outside the context of an anxiety disorder, has been associated with higher risk for suicide.

Psychotic disorders

The presence of psychosis contributes to more than 10% of suicides, and schizophrenia is associated with a tenfold increased risk of death by suicide. Studies have shown that up to 50% of schizophrenia patients may attempt suicide at some point in the course of their illness. Suicide attempts in schizophrenia are frequently precipitated by depression, psychosocial stressors and psychotic symptoms, are often medically serious, and are often associated with a high degree of intent.

Suicide in schizophrenia is most common during the early years following illness onset, and an increased risk of suicide has been correlated with a number of factors, including patient attributes, symptom characteristics and period in illness course. Patients at higher risk for suicide include those who have a chronic unremitting illness course, those who have required multiple psychiatric hospitalizations and those who have made a previous suicide attempt. In addition, patients with significant depressive symptoms, patients with good premorbid functioning and patients who understand or have insight into the implications of having a chronic psychotic illness (those who appreciate the negative impact of the illness on their personal, social and vocational functioning and achievement, and those who recognize a loss of previous skills and competencies) are also at high risk, particularly if they are pessimistic about the benefits of treatment. Other factors associated with increased suicide risk include male gender, younger age, social isolation, severe agitation or akathisia (substantive subjective restlessness) and the presence of prominent positive psychotic symptoms. Patients who feel terrorized by their symptoms, those experiencing persecutory delusions and those experiencing aggressive or suicidal command hallucinations may be at particularly high risk for self-injurious behaviours and completed suicide (the presence of prominent negative psychotic symptoms, such as apathy and avolition, is associated with a reduced risk of suicide).

Command hallucinations are auditory hallucinations that instruct the individual to perform specific actions, think specific thoughts or behave in specific ways. Not all command-type hallucinations necessarily pose a safety issue for the patient. For example, command hallucinations that instruct the patient to close a door or wear a particular colour of clothing are benign (although they may be distressing to the patient). On the other hand, command hallucinations that instruct the patient to engage in risk-taking behaviours, to harm themselves or to harm others may be lethal! It is difficult to predict which patients are more or less likely to obey command hallucinations; thus, any patient who is experiencing dangerous command hallucinations should be closely monitored.

For many patients the period immediately following discharge from hospital and periods of improvement after relapse confer the highest risk for suicide or suicide attempts. This may be partly attributable to the improved insight that often accompanies symptom improvement, which may allow patients to appreciate: the impact of the illness on their ability to function in and be accepted by society; the loss of previous skills, relationships and social position; and the consequences of the stigmatization of and discrimination against the mentally ill. In addition, the onset of postpsychotic depression following an acute episode has been identified as a vulnerable time for patients with schizophrenia, particularly young males with good insight and good premorbid functioning.

Factors that may increase suicide risk in schizophrenia
- insight into deficits caused by illness
- self-harm/violent command hallucinations
- akathisia – may be related to side effects of antipsychotic medications
- agitation – may be related to side effects of antipsychotic medications
- depressive symptoms
- feelings of hopelessness
- social stress – variably financial difficulties
- recent hospital discharge
- social isolation
- male gender
- age less than 45 years.

Personality disorders

According to a number of studies, having a personality disorder, particularly a borderline or antisocial personality disorder, may be a

Summary of risk factors associated with psychiatric history

Psychiatric disorders associated with increased suicide risk	Higher risk	Lower risk
Major depressive disorder	Hopelessness	Absence of acute episode of mental disorder
Bipolar disorder (depressive or mixed episode)	Severe depression	
	Acute psychosis	Treated mental illness
Substance-use disorder	Substance abuse	
Anxiety disorder	Noncompliance	Supportive environment
Schizophrenia	Poorly controlled symptoms	Compliance with treatment
Personality disorders (particularly borderline personality disorder)		Low substance use

factor in up to 5% of suicides. Lifetime rates of suicide for these disorders range from 3 to 9%. Rates of both self-harm behaviours and suicide attempts are high in this patient population. The presence of acute psychosocial stress or crisis increases the risk in this group.

Psychiatric symptoms

Specific cognitive, affective and behavioural symptoms, within or outside the context of a psychiatric disorder, have been independently associated with increased suicide risk.

Cognitive symptoms associated with increased suicide risk
- suicide ideation
- hopelessness
- low self-esteem
- cognitive and social skills deficits – poor coping and problem-solving skills, rigid thinking, cognitive distortions
- psychosis – particularly command hallucinations regarding self-harm or safety
- intoxication.

Affective symptoms associated with increased suicide risk
- depressed mood
- affective states that are poorly controlled, intense, severe and poorly tolerated:
  - anger
  - dysphoria
  - guilt
  - anxiety
  - tension
  - panic states

Summary of psychiatric symptoms that may increase suicide risk

Psychiatric symptoms associated with increased suicide risk	Higher risk	Lower risk
Cognitive symptoms	Hopelessness Decreased self-esteem Cognitive skills deficits Command hallucinations Intoxication	Positive self-esteem Cognitive flexibility Good coping strategies and problem-solving skills Future focus Optimism Religiosity
Affective symptoms	Depressed mood Severe anhedonia Severe anxiety/panic attacks Intense, poorly tolerated affective states	Ability to manage emotion and tolerate negative affective states
Behavioural symptoms	Behavioural activation Severe insomnia Impulsivity Aggression Akathisia Alcohol and substance misuse	Ability to self-sooth Good self-control

    o fearfulness
    o loneliness
    o shame
    o humiliation
- severe anhedonia – the loss of capacity to experience pleasure.

Behavioural symptoms associated with increased suicide risk
- behavioural activation – restlessness, agitation, insomnia
- severe insomnia
- impulsivity
- poor self-control
- unconstrained aggressive behaviour
- akathisia – substantial subjective restlessness, often attributable to a medication side effect
- alcohol and substance misuse.

Medical history

Patients who have recently been diagnosed with a life-threatening or progressive chronic illness or an illness that would bring severe humiliation and shame to them in their sociocultural context may be at increased risk for suicide, particularly if the reaction to the diagnosis is severe and the patient lacks social supports.

Physical illness associated with functional impairment, cognitive impairment, pain, disfigurement, increased dependence on others, and decreases in vision or hearing are associated with increased risk of suicide. Neurological disorders such as epilepsy, multiple sclerosis, Huntington disease, and brain and spinal-cord injury are associated with a particularly high risk for suicide.

Other physical disorders that have been found to be associated with an increased risk for suicide include the following:
- human immunodeficiency virus (HIV)/acquired immunodeficiency syndrome (AIDS)
- malignancies
- peptic ulcer disease
- systemic lupus erythematosus
- chronic haemodialysis-treated renal failure

- heart disease
- chronic obstructive pulmonary disease
- prostate disease.

The risk for suicide or suicide attempts in the context of physical illness is highly correlated with the presence of a psychiatric illness (particularly depression) or psychiatric symptoms (such as hopelessness), as well as with the individual patient's personality and coping style, the availability of social supports, the presence of psychosocial stressors and any previous history of suicidal behaviours. In addition, the meaning and consequences of the illness to the patient are an important consideration in estimating risk.

Although rates of depression are increased in those with serious medical illness, depression is not a logical or expected outcome of having a chronic or life-threatening disease (most people with chronic or life-threatening diseases may have depressed or despondent feelings but will not develop clinical depression). When clinical depression does occur in a person with a chronic or life-threatening disease, it must be appropriately treated and the individual must be evaluated for suicidal ideas, intentions and plans. Depression and associated suicidal ideation tend to be underdetected and undertreated in the medically ill.

Characteristics of medical history associated with increased suicide risk

- recent diagnoses of life-threatening illness
- chronic illness
- neurological disorders
- illness associated with:
  - severe insomnia
  - unremitting, chronic pain
  - functional impairment
  - cognitive impairment
  - loss of sight or hearing
  - disfigurement
  - perceived burdensomeness
  - hopelessness regarding prognosis
  - presence of psychiatric disorder
  - presence of psychiatric symptoms
  - shame and humiliation.

Increased suicidality in HIV/AIDS may be associated with the following:

- presence of HIV dementia (often characterized by labile mood, behavioural disinhibition, impaired judgment, impulsivity)
- presence of a psychiatric disorder
- substance abuse
- previous suicide attempts
- depression
- greater number of disease symptoms
- loneliness
- need for support
- younger age
- current stressors (unemployment, bereavement, etc.)
- poor adaptive functioning
- hopelessness
- internalizing pattern.

Summary of medical history risk factors

Medical disorders associated with increased risk	Higher risk	Lower risk
Recent diagnoses of life-threatening illness	Severe insomnia	Disease remission
	Unremitting, chronic pain	Feeling physically well
	Cognitive impairment	Acceptance
Chronic illness	Loss of sight or hearing	Good social supports
Neurological disorders	Functional impairment	
	Perceived burdensomeness	
	Disfigurement	
	Hopelessness regarding prognosis	
	Presence of psychiatric disorder	
	Presence of psychiatric symptoms	
	Shame and humiliation	

Family history

A number of factors in the family history influence the risk for suicidal behaviours and completed suicide. Both a history of suicide (particularly in first-degree relatives) and a history of psychiatric illness in the family confer increased risk. In addition, history of family violence, abuse or neglect is associated with higher risk.

Question

What about genetics and biology?

Answer

Genetic factors may also play a role. Monozygotic (identical) twins have a significantly higher rate of both completed suicide and suicide attempts than do dizygotic (nonidentical or fraternal) twins. Adoption studies following children who have been raised by their biological families and comparing them with adopted-away children raised by adoptive families have shown that suicide rates of adopted-away children are comparable with those of their biological families rather than their adopted families.

A number of biological factors have also been associated with suicide. For example, neurobiological studies have found reduced levels of serotonin metabolites (5-hydroxyindoleacetic acid) in the CNS fluid of adult suicide victims. Serotonin is a brain neurochemical implicated in the regulation of mood and cognition. Abnormalities of brain serotonin function have been demonstrated in patients who suffer from a variety of psychiatric illnesses, most notably depression. More recently, increases in the numbers of brain serotonin receptor 2A (5-HT2A) and genetic abnormalities of the serotonin system (polymorphism of the serotonin 2 receptor gene) have been described. These seem to be independent of the serotonin abnormalities found in depression without suicide.

Studies have also suggested an alteration in the hypothalamic–pituitary–adrenal axis in individuals at risk for suicide and in the growth hormone response to the chemical apomorphine. Additionally, research into neurotrophins (molecules important in brain synaptic plasticity and in the maintenance and growth of nerve cells) has identified abnormalities in a number of these compounds (such as brain-derived neurotrophic factor (BDNF), neurotrophin 3 (NT- 3) and nerve growth factor (NGF)) in specific brain regions (the hippocampus and the prefrontal cortex) in successful suicides. Gene expression studies of post mortem brain tissue suggest biological differences in those who commit suicide even when controlling for the presence of a depressive disorder.

Taken as a whole, these studies suggest that there is a relationship between the neurotransmitter systems involved in depression and suicide but that individuals who commit suicide may have additional underlying genetic vulnerabilities that increase their risk. This research is still in its infancy and it is not currently possible to identify which individuals may carry this enhanced genetic risk.

Summary of family history risk factors

Family history associated with increased suicide risk	Higher risk	Lower risk
Suicide	Suicide in a first-degree relative	No family history of suicide
Mental disorder	Mental illness in a first-degree relative	No family history of mental illness

Personal history

A patient's personal history includes the circumstances and socio-cultural, political and financial context into which the person is born. It includes the person's emotional, psychological, social and physical growth and development. It also includes a person's school, work and social adjustment and functioning as well as an understanding of current and past significant life events and psychosocial stressors.

Early negative environmental factors, such as an impoverished environment and early exposure to trauma, neglect and abuse, are associated with increased suicide risk. Suicide rates are increased at least 10-fold in those with a history of childhood sexual or physical abuse. Individuals living in deprived areas, those with lower educational levels, financial difficulties or legal difficulties, and those who are unemployed have also been found to be at higher risk for suicide.

Persons living in deprived areas are more likely to have decreased access to appropriate health care, education, employment opportunities and social services and supports. For some individuals, unemployment can be associated with a number of other factors that may increase suicide risk. For example, loss of employment may translate into loss of financial and family security, loss of residence, and significant interpersonal, marital and emotional stress. Alternatively, unemployment, job loss or failure to gain and maintain employment may reflect other issues such as the loss of skills and capabilities consequent to a physical or psychiatric disorder; alcohol- or substance-use problems; the presence of maladaptive personality traits that are disruptive to the workplace or interfere with working with others; the presence of psychosocial circumstances associated with stigma and discrimination; poverty; lack of schooling or vocational training; and domestic violence or abuse. Thus the relationship between unemployment and suicide may be bidirectional.

Low socioeconomic status, poverty and loss of financial security have been identified as significant proximal risk factors for suicide particularly in eastern countries. The suicide story in agricultural areas in India is one example of the incredible toll that economic and political factors can have on communities and families. In 2009 alone, 1500 farmers committed suicide after being forced into debt in one of India's agricultural states.

Question

Does the type of employment influence suicide risk?

Answer

Health care professionals, particularly physicians and dentists, appear to be at higher risk of suicide compared with other professional groups. The reason for this is unknown.

The presence or absence of social and emotional supports plays an important part in the estimation of suicide risk. Whereas the presence of a strong social support system may reduce suicide risk, the absence of a support system, living alone and social isolation can significantly increase the risk for suicide. The presence and involvement of family, friends and meaningful others in an individual's life has a powerful protective influence against the risk for both completed suicide and suicide attempts.

Being married, or in a long-term committed partnership, may be protective against suicide, although the nature of the relationship must be considered. Individuals in dysfunctional or conflictual relationship may be more likely to have a higher rather than a lower risk for suicide. As noted in the discussion above regarding gender and suicide risk, domestic violence and abuse are associated with increased risk of suicide. The risk for suicide attempts in individuals who have experienced recent domestic partner violence is four- to eightfold higher than the risk for individuals without such experiences.

This notwithstanding, the suicide rate among single adults is twice that of married adults, and rates among those who are divorced, separated or widowed are four to five times higher than those for married individuals. However, it is not possible to determine if this is a cause-and-effect relationship. Are people who are less prone to suicide able to create and hold long-term intimate relationships or does the presence of a long-term intimate relationship mitigate suicide, or both?

For individuals with strong affiliation to traditional values, cultures and family systems, suicide risk may be strongly influenced by cultural, religious, social and family dynamic factors, regardless of whether the person is living within or outside the family's place of cultural heritage. Although data from Eastern countries is limited, studies are now quickly emerging that shed new light on proximal risk factors influencing suicide risk. Domestic problems including marital problems, financial problems, conflict with in-laws, forced marriage, unwanted pregnancy, emotional, physical or sexual abuse, familial alcohol misuse, and other family problems have been identified as strong proximal triggers for suicide attempts in woman in China,

Sri Lanka, Pakistan and India. Suicide in these contexts is most often impulsive and most cases are not associated with a diagnosable psychiatric disorder.

There is often a 'trigger' – a stressor or precipitating event – linked to a suicide death. This trigger is superimposed on proximal and distal risk factors that must be understood together in the context of an individual's life. Interpersonal loss is a commonly associated proximal trigger for suicide death and suicide behaviour. Loss may be real, as in the death of a loved one, or perceived, as in the threatened loss of a relationship. Other proximal triggers may include interpersonal conflict, rejection, loss of employment, economic problems, legal problems and eviction. As noted above, physical illness associated with functional impairments, cognitive impairment, depression, pain, disfigurement, loss of independence and neurological deficits such as loss in vision or hearing may also be proximal triggers. The medical diagnoses most closely associated with increased suicide risk include cancer, HIV/AIDS and neurological disorders.

Exposure to 'suicide', whether directly – through the loss of a close friend or family member to suicide – or indirectly – through media and other sources – can also increase risk. Media reporting and portrayal of suicide and suicidal behaviour can influence suicide and self-harm in the general population. Newspaper reporting of suicides can be particularly influential if it is sensational, if it includes dramatic headlines and pictures, if it reports methods of suicide in detail, and if the subject is a celebrity. There are numerous examples of 'copycat' suicides that follow widespread media coverage of suicides. Evidence of media influences on suicide has led to the development and promotion of guidelines for the reporting and portrayal of suicide behaviour. Implementation of media guidelines and the portrayal of suicide within communities and families, however, is strongly influenced by social and cultural attitudes, beliefs, and the meaning ascribed to a suicide death. Cultures and families can inadvertently, overtly or covertly condone suicide as a solution to deal with shame, humiliation, physical illness, the failure of a marriage, the loss of social position, bereavement or other psychosocial crisis. The romantic portrayal of the 'Romeo and Juliet' type of suicide is one such example. Another is the glorification of suicide committed as an act of martyrdom, such as self-inflicted death committed as a declaration of religious devotion, nationalism or political belief.

Repeated exposure to suicide, whether through stories depicted in the news, on television, in movies, on the internet, or through personal experience with the suicide of a family member or friend, may increase suicide risk through a process of habituation. Over time, repeated exposure to 'suicide' may make suicide more permissive, lead to reduced fear of suicide behaviour, and lead to acceptance of suicide as a normalized response to crisis or distress.

Question

Does sexual orientation or choice of intimate partner influence suicide risk?

Answer

There is an insufficient number of appropriately controlled studies currently available to specifically answer this question. However, homosexual, bisexual and transgendered individuals are at higher risk for a variety of health, mental health and social problems, including depression, substance abuse, social exclusion, homelessness, sexual risk-taking, sexually transmitted diseases, poor health maintenance and school dropout. Studies involving diverse populations do suggest that homosexual or bisexual individuals are at higher risk for suicide attempts, particularly gay and lesbian youth; however, there is no evidence that the rates of completed suicide are higher than that of the general population.

Suicide risk factors for this group may include cultural attitudes, stigma and discrimination against gays and lesbians, stress related to disclosure of sexual orientation to friends and family, gender nonconformity, and aggression against homosexuals. Youth who are struggling with issues of homosexuality and become concurrently clinically depressed may be at higher risk for a suicide attempt or death by suicide.

Summary of psychosocial history risk factors

Psychosocial history associated with increased suicide risk	Higher risk	Lower risk
Lack of social support	Divorced or widowed	Married
Unemployment	Unemployed	Employed
Drop in socioeconomic status	Conflictual interpersonal relationships	Stable relationships
Family discord	Low personal achievement	Children in the home
Domestic violence	Social isolation	Good achievement
Recent stressful life event	Poor interpersonal relationships	Positive social support
Childhood sexual/ physical abuse	Domestic violence	Positive therapeutic relationship
	Sexual abuse	Absence of abuse
	Physical abuse	Supportive family

Personality

A person's 'life view' and the way they relate to and interact with their environment are important factors influencing how they will respond to adversity. There is no 'suicidal' personality, but a patient's individual personality traits, ability to manage emotional and psychological pain, problem-solving skills, past responses to stress and ability to use internal and external resources during crises are important factors that may mitigate or increase risk for suicide. Individuals who are impulsive, reactionary, feel they are not able to make change (have a poor sense of self-efficacy), have difficulty problem-solving and seeking alternative solutions, and lack healthy coping strategies to deal with life adversity may be at higher risk for suicide. Healthy and well-developed coping skills help buffer stressful live events and allow individuals to access internal and external resources during crises.

In terms of personality, suicide risk may be associated with hostile, helpless, dependent and rigid personality traits. Individuals at higher risk of suicide may include those with rigid 'all or none' thinking. These individuals often have difficulty in problem-solving during times of stress. Even if they are ambivalent about suicide they may see suicide as their only option because they are unable to come up with alternative strategies. In addition, individuals who are perfectionistic with excessively high personal expectations may be at higher risk for suicide, particularly in the context of perceived failure or humiliation. Individuals who have an enduring hopeless, fatalistic or pessimistic approach to life may also be at higher risk.

Summary of personality risk factors

Personality features associated with increased suicide risk	Higher risk	Lower risk
Cognitive and social-skills deficits	Poor coping skills	Good insight
Pessimism	Poor problem-solving skills	Sense of responsibility to family
Hopelessness	Poor insight	Good reality-testing
Perfectionism	Rigid thinking	Positive coping skills
Rigid or black-and-white thinking	Poor stress tolerance	Positive problem-solving skills
	Poor self-regulation	Flexibility
	Poor emotional control	Ability to manage emotion/affect

By knowing these risk factors, will I be able to prevent all patients from committing suicide?

Unfortunately, the answer is 'no'. No specific risk factor or set of risk factors has been identified that is consistently predictive of suicide or other suicidal behaviours.

Identification of 'suicide risk factors' does not allow a completely accurate prediction of when or if a specific individual will in fact die by suicide.

Thus, suicide assessment scales that rely on the cataloguing of patient risk factors, although a useful clinical aid in the assessment of suicide risk, cannot by themselves be used successfully to predict who will commit suicide. They can, however, give the clinician an idea of how significant the total risk load may be and thus flag those individuals for whom preventive interventions should be immediately initiated. Thus, a scale such as the Tool for Assessment of Suicide Risk (TASR) (see Chapter 4 and Appendix A) can be a useful tool in the clinical evaluation of patients. Additionally, risk factors when taken together to identify the 'burden' of risk are most useful in addressing proximal rather than distal events. Accurately predicting the future is difficult enough. Accurately predicting the distant future may not be possible.

What can be done?

Remember: Most patients who experience suicidal thoughts or engage in suicide behaviours will not die by suicide. Most will choose life rather than death.

As discussed in the introduction, suicide is complex and is influenced by innumerable underlying factors. Some of these factors will respond to appropriately targeted interventions. This is particularly true of those individuals who may be suffering from a mental disorder. Health professionals can ensure that each patient receives a thorough clinical evaluation, with attention given to the patient's current presentation, individual strengths and weaknesses, history and psychosocial situation. This information can then be used to estimate the patient's suicide risk, with the primary goal of reducing that risk and thereby reducing the likelihood of death by suicide. Identification and treatment of an existing mental disorder, for example, can significantly reduce individual suicide risk.

Summary of suicide risk factors

Area of risk assessment	Higher risk	Lower risk
Age		
Elderly	Elderly	Prepubertal
Youth	15–35 years	
Adult		
Gender		
Male	Male	Female
Female		
Women	Intimate partner abuse	Pregnancy
	Domestic violence and abuse	Young children in the home
	Postpartum depression (PPD)	Strong sense of responsibility to family
	Postpartum psychosis (PPP)	
	Rigid role expectations	
	Institutionalized gender inequality	
Suicidality		
Suicide ideation	Persistent	Fleeting
	Intense	Low-intensity
	Uncontrollable	Manageable
	Acute	
	Prolonged	
Suicide intent	Strong desire to die	High ambivalence
	Strong commitment to act	Low commitment to act
	Expectation of death	
Suicide plans	Premeditated	No plan
	Well-planned	Choice of low lethality
	Highly lethal means	No access to means
	Access to means	

(continued)

(*Continued*)

Area of risk assessment	Higher risk	Lower risk
Method lethality	Firearm Hanging Jumping Pesticide poisoning	Overdose
Past suicide behaviours (PSB)		
Detected suicide attempts	Recent attempt	First attempt
Undetected suicide attempts	Multiple past attempts	
Aborted suicide attempts		
Self-harm behaviours		
Context of PSB	Low chance of discovery	High chance of rescue
Consequences of PSB	Serious adverse consequences	
Intent of PSB	High intent to die	Low intent
Planning of PSB	Premeditated and well-planned	
Method of PSB	Use of highly lethal means	Low-lethality method
Feelings about PSB	Regret of survival	Grateful for survival Regret of attempt High ambivalence
Psychiatric disorders		
Major depressive disorder	Hopelessness Severe depression	Remission or recovery
Bipolar disorder	Depressive phase of bipolar disorder	Absence of acute distressing
Substance-use disorder		symptoms
Anxiety disorder	Mixed phase of bipolar disorder	Treated mental illness
Schizophrenia	Acute psychosis	Supportive environment Compliance with treatment

(Continued)

Area of risk assessment	Higher risk	Lower risk
Personality disorders	Substance abuse Noncompliance Poorly controlled symptoms Borderline personality disorder	Low substance use
Psychiatric symptoms		
Cognitive symptoms	Hopelessness Poor self-esteem Cognitive skills deficits Poor reality-testing Command hallucinations Intoxication	Intact reality-testing Good coping strategies and problem-solving skills Ability to manage emotion and tolerate negative affective states Future focus Religiosity
Affective symptoms	Depressed mood Severe anhedonia Severe anxiety/fear/ panic attacks Intense anger Intense shame and humiliation Intense loneliness	Mild mood symptoms Stable Tolerated
Behavioural symptoms	Behavioural activation Impulsivity Aggression Akathisia Alcohol and substance misuse	Ability to self-sooth Good self-control Low substance use

(continued)

(*Continued*)

Area of risk assessment	Higher risk	Lower risk
Medical history		
Recent diagnoses of life-threatening illness	Severe insomnia	Disease remission
	Unremitting, chronic pain	Feeling physically well
Chronic illness	Functional impairment	Good adjustment
Neurological disorders	Cognitive impairment	Acceptance
	Loss of sight or hearing	Good social supports
	Disfigurement	
	Perceived burdensomeness	
	Hopelessness	
	Comorbid psychiatric disorder	
	Comorbid psychiatric symptoms	
	Shame and humiliation	
Family history		
Suicide	Suicide in immediate family	No family history of suicide
Mental disorder	Mental illness in immediate family	No family history of mental illness
Personal history		
Social isolation	Living alone	Married
Poor-quality relationships	Poor infrastructure of support	Positive social support
Domestic conflict	Divorced or widowed	Stable relationships
Life stressors	Poor-quality relationships	Supportive family
Significant losses		Children in the home

(Continued)

Area of risk assessment	Higher risk	Lower risk
Recent stressful life event	Conflictual/unstable relationships	Absence of abuse
Childhood sexual/ physical abuse	Domestic violence and abuse	Employed
	Legal problems	Good achievement
	Financial problems	
	Unemployed	
	Loss of employment	
	Loss of status	
	Loss of relationship	
	Bereavement	
	Loss of health	
	Loss of function/ disability	
	Low personal achievement	
Personality		
Cognitive and social skills deficits	Poor coping skills	Insightful
Pessimism	Poor problem-solving skills Poor insight	Sense of responsibility to family
Hopelessness	Rigid thinking	Good reality-testing
Perfectionism	Poor stress tolerance	Positive coping skills
Rigid or black-and-white thinking	Poor self-regulation	Positive problem-solving skills
	Poor emotional control	Flexibility
		Able to manage emotion/affect

Chapter 3
Suicide Risk Assessment

Introduction

The goals of the suicide risk assessment are to identify and understand the relevance of the suicide risk and protective factors for an individual patient in order to estimate the level (low, moderate, high) of suicide risk and to inform clinical decision-making regarding immediate safety management and the development of targeted immediate, short-term and long-term interventions.

Question

Who needs an assessment?

Answer

Although some of the risk factors previously discussed may be of limited utility in identifying which individuals will or will not commit suicide, these risk factors can be useful in identifying who must receive an assessment. Remember that individual risk factors can be proximal or distal to the onset of suicidal behaviours and no risk factor taken alone necessarily increases or decreases risk. It is the weighting and confluence of specific suicide risk factors rather than the number of risk factors present that must be considered in determining risk, and the relevance of risk factors must be understood from within the psychosocial-cultural context and life experience of each individual patient.

Suicide Risk Management: A Manual for Health Professionals, Second Edition.
Sonia Chehil and Stan Kutcher.
© 2012 John Wiley & Sons, Ltd. Published 2012 by John Wiley & Sons, Ltd.

Any patient presenting with depressive symptoms, any individual who has made a suicide attempt or engaged in other self-harm behaviours, and any individual who expresses suicidal thoughts and/or hopelessness should be assessed as soon as possible. Those who engage in self-destructive behaviours, such as self-mutilation (cutting, burning), should also be assessed because such behaviours may be motivated by underlying suicidal thoughts or plans and may be an expression of an underlying mental disorder.

Patients who present in crisis or who have experienced a recent traumatic event or loss (whether actual or perceived) should always be assessed for suicide risk. Attempts to understand the patient's experience from their perspective is important. Subjective experiences of similar events are highly variable. For example, the death of a relative may be devastating to one individual but have minimal impact on another. Similarly, for some individuals anticipated or perceived loss may be as stressful as actual loss. For example, to some, the threat of loss of a relationship can be as overwhelming as the experience of actual termination of the relationship. Likewise, what is experienced as shame or humiliation and how shame and humiliation are addressed reflect a myriad of individual, social, and cultural factors. Understanding what an experience means to the individual, taking into account their familial, cultural and social context, can provide important insights into the personal relevance and subsequent weighting of experiences in the evaluation of suicide risk.

Patients who have recently been diagnosed with a life-threatening or progressive chronic illness or an illness that will bring them severe humiliation and shame, and those who are suffering from illnesses associated with unremitting chronic pain, loss of function and perceived sense of being or becoming a 'burden' on loved ones should be assessed periodically for suicide risk, particularly during times of illness exacerbation. In addition, patients suffering from a medical illness who express hopelessness regarding their prognosis and those who experience accompanying psychiatric symptoms should be periodically assessed for suicide risk.

Any patient with a psychiatric illness should be evaluated for suicide risk at baseline and periodically throughout their illness course, regardless of their clinical status.

Question

For patients suffering from a mental disorder, when should an evaluation for suicide risk be performed?

Answer

There are particular times in the patient's illness course that may be associated with higher suicide risk and call for a higher index of suspicion on the part of the health care provider. For patients with mental illness, suicide risk **must** be evaluated:

- At the initial baseline assessment.
- During periods of heightened stress or crisis.
- When a change in patient observation status or treatment setting is contemplated. For example, prior to discharging any patient from an inpatient unit, prior to changing patient hospital privileges (for example, discontinuation of one-on-one observation or provision of patient passes outside of hospital) and on discharging patients from the emergency room setting.
- When there is a sudden change in clinical presentation. Any patient who experiences a sudden decompensation or worsening in their symptoms must be assessed for suicide risk. Any patient who experiences a sudden unexpected improvement in symptoms must also be assessed for suicide risk. Some patients, particularly those suffering from depressive illness, may feel a sense of relief and joy after making the decision to end their life. Death may be a welcome escape from what is perceived and experienced as endless suffering and unremitting pain. To some, the decision to choose death by suicide may symbolize regaining of control over their lives and releasing of the burden of their illness. To others, death may be seen as a way to reunite with lost loved ones, to reach utopia or to experience a rebirth into a better life.
- When there is failure to experience improvement or a worsening of symptoms despite treatment.

Learning how to assess suicide risk

- Step I Being prepared
- Step II Identifying 'warning signs' of suicide risk
- Step III Evaluating current suicidality
- Step IV Evaluating past suicide behaviours
- Step V Evaluating suicide risk and protective factors
- Step VI Identifying what's going on
- Step VII Identifying targets for intervention

Step I Being prepared

It is important for clinicians to explore their own feelings, beliefs and attitudes about suicide and self-harm and to be aware of how working with suicidal patients may affect them emotionally, personally and professionally. Being confronted with patients who are at risk for suicide or who have attempted suicide can be stressful even for the most seasoned clinician. Clinicians may experience a variety of reactions when working with a suicidal patient, including feelings of helplessness, anger, anxiety, disappointment, ambivalence, sadness, ineptitude or rejection. Whether in a community office, in the accident and emergency department or in another location, a clinician's reactions to or feelings about a suicidal patient and/or about suicide in general can influence their ability to perform an objective professional assessment of risk and can influence their clinical decision-making regarding care and treatment. Being prepared to work with patients at risk for suicide requires development of skills to effectively manage these emotions. It is equally important that clinicians prepare themselves for the possibility that some patients at risk for suicide will die by suicide and that they accept that not all suicides can be prevented, despite the best efforts of the health care team.

Health providers practising outside of the hospital or accident and emergency setting must also be prepared to initiate or access immediate emergency support and intervention for patients who present after having initiated a suicide plan or made a suicide attempt. This is a

suicide in process and is a **medical emergency**. All health providers should be prepared to provide emergency first aid management and know what to do, who to call, where to go and how to get there in order to maximize the patient's chance for survival.

Being prepared can assist the health provider in providing the highest quality of care to suicidal patients:

1 Be aware of your own thoughts and feelings about suicide and suicidal patients.

2 Accept that suicide is not always preventable.

3 Develop healthy strategies to effectively manage harmful emotional, psychological and behavioural reactions to the suicidal patient.

4 Be prepared emotionally, psychologically, personally and professionally for the death of a patient by suicide.

5 Talk to colleagues who work with high-risk patients about how they cope with and manage working with suicidal patients and how they have coped with and managed the death of a patient by suicide.

6 Be aware of the supports available to you if and when you may need them.

7 Be confident in your ability to assess and manage suicide risk:

a Know the 'warning signs' of acute suicide risk.

b Know the suicide risk and protective factors.

c Know the unique risk factors relevant to the populations you serve.

d Know how to ask patients about suicidality.

e Know how to determine suicide risk.

f Know how to manage suicide risk.

g Consult with peers for support, to debrief, for case reviews, and to discuss clinical decision-making and case management.

h Know the services and supports available for patients in your jurisdiction and how these supports and services can be accessed.

i Know the laws governing consent, confidentiality, release of information and involuntary hospital admission in your jurisdiction.

8 Be prepared to initiate or access immediate emergency management if confronted with a suicide in process.

Asking about suicide and suicide behaviours and trying to understand triggers and risk factors for suicide can be awkward and difficult. Integrating this type of inquiry into the standard or traditional medical evaluation by clinicians who are not accustomed to asking these questions or in settings where this type of inquiry has not generally been performed takes practice. Establishing rapport with the patient involves active listening and is the initial approach to any medical assessment, but particularly one involving a patient who presents with suicidality (suicidal ideas, suicide plan or a suicidal attempt). Use of a calm, patient, nonjudgemental and empathic approach will help in developing rapport with the patient.

General active listening tips to use during the assessment:
- Maintain a comfortable body position:
  o Make sure you are a comfortable distance from the patient.
  o Sit a little to the side – not directly in front of the patient.
  o Keep your posture relaxed.
  o Lean forward slightly.
- Maintain a calm, involved and neutral facial expression
- Maintain positive eye contact that demonstrates interest, curiosity and caring:
  o This varies across cultures so adapt to your population.
  o Don't avoid eye contact but DON'T STARE!
- Keep focused on the patient.
- Use verbal and nonverbal communication to encourage the patient to share:
  o Gestures like **nodding**.
  o Words like **'Okay'**, **'Sure'**, **'Right'**, **'Uh-huh'**.
  o Phrases like **'I get it'**, **'Tell me more'**, **'Please continue'**, **'I hear you'**.

Beginning your assessment with empathic, nonthreatening statements followed by gentle enquiry is a good way to ease into the assessment.

The following are some examples of how this discussion could be initiated.

The empathic statement
- 'I can see how difficult things have been for you lately...'
- 'It seems that things have been hard for you and that it has been difficult to cope...'
- 'You seem to be having a hard time...'

The gentle enquiry
- 'Help me understand how this has been for you.'
- 'Can you share your concerns with me?'
- 'Tell me about what has been happening.'
- 'How have things been for you lately?'

Step II Identifying 'warning signs' of suicide risk

Remember that suicidality can be overt or covert – concealed. Being aware of possible 'warning signs' for both active and concealed suicidality is essential for the early detection and evaluation of patients at high risk for suicide.

Warning signs of suicidality

The presence of suicidality – suicide ideation, intent or plan – attempted suicide or self-harm behaviour confers **acute risk** and signals the need for a thorough suicide risk assessment. Warning signs of suicidality include: threatening to self-harm or commit suicide; talking or writing about death, dying or suicide; seeking means to self-hurt or commit suicide; making preparations for dying – such as preparing a will, giving away possessions, saying goodbye to loved ones, making reparations in relationships.

Additional factors or warning signs that signal the need for an immediate and thorough suicide risk assessment include the following:
- Patients in acute or extreme distress or who are experiencing affective states that are intense, severe or intolerable (anger, despair, shame, guilt, humiliation, loneliness, fear).
- Patients with current, evolving or anticipated personal or psycho-social crisis.
- Patients who are feeling hopeless, trapped by their problems or that there is no reason for living.

Warning signs of concealed suicidality

Sometimes a person contemplating suicide reaches out to a health provider but does not know how to make the clinician aware of their distress. For example: the young man who comes to the emergency room with no obvious physical injury or acute physical health problem; the middle aged executive who seems 'depressed' and frequently seeks medical care about vague health complaints; the elderly woman whose spouse has recently died and who is 'drinking a little too much'. When faced with these or similar out-of-the-usual circumstances, consider the possibility of concealed suicidality.

Suspect concealed suicidality in patients who present with profound social withdrawal, intense negative affective states (despair, shame, humiliation, anger, rage, disgrace, fear), psychosis, irrational thinking; those who seem distart or disconnect; those who avoid or refuse to answer questions about suicidality or who provide value or cryptric responses; those who express hopelessness or worthlessness.

What to do?

1 Look for 'warning signs' of possible conealed suicidal ideation, intent or plan:

   a Is there any evidence of psychosis?

   b Are you unable to develop rapport with the individual?

   c Is the patient reluctant to answer direct questions about suicidality?

   d Does the patient respond with 'I don't know' to questions about suicidality?

   e Is the patient giving you nonverbal clues that raise suspicion of underlying suicidality:
   - Does the patient appear despondent or emotionally distant?
   - Does the patient appear angry or agitated?
   - Is the patient restless?
   - Is the patient avoiding eye contact?

   f Is the patient giving you verbal clues that are incongruent with the patient's presentation or that point to there being more going on than is being disclosed:
   - 'I can't do this anymore.'
   - 'I can't cope.'

- 'There's nothing you can do.'
- 'I'm fine.'
- 'It doesn't matter.'

2 Look for evidence of past suicidality in the patient's hospital records (e.g. past suicide attempts and suspicious injuries that may have been unreported attempts) or during the physical exam (e.g. scars from self-inflicted lacerations).

3 Complete the suicide risk assessment even if much of the information is not available.

4 Place particular emphasis on the evaluation of current high-risk psychiatric symptoms and on uncovering the presence of a possible psychiatric disorder that may place the individual at high risk.

5 Err on the side of caution when making decisions regarding disposition and intervention . . . If your gut says something is not right, something is probably not right!

Step III Evaluating current suicidality

The evaluation of current suicidality includes the assessment of the following areas:

1 **Triggers for suicidality**   Acute precipitating factors for suicide thoughts, behaviours and actions.

2 **Suicide ideation**   Recent and immediate frequency, intensity and duration of suicide thoughts.

3 **Suicide intent**   Recent and immediate expectation and commitment to die.

4 **Suicide plans**   Method, availability, belief in lethality, chance of rescue and preparation.

5 **Suicide motivation**   Personal meaning and drive to die.

6 **Suicide buffers**   Reasons for living and internal strengths for managing risk.

Unfortunately, some people who are contemplating suicide may be reluctant to reveal suicidal thoughts, intent or plans to a health care provider even when asked directly. They may be even less likely to reveal suicidal thoughts to a clinician with whom they do not have a therapeutic relationship. Failure to disclose substantive suicidal thoughts is a particularly pertinent issue for clinicians in casualty departments, where they are often faced with having to assess suicide risk in those whom they are meeting for the first time.

Providing an introductory statement that 'normalizes' the experience of suicide thoughts, intent or plans can help the patient feel more comfortable about the clinician's upcoming line of inquiry. Once the patient feels comfortable in the interview situation they are more likely to disclose thoughts and plans about suicide to the clinician.

The 'normalizing' introductory statement

'I can see that you have been having a difficult time ... Sometimes when people are going through things, such as those that you have just shared with me, they have thoughts that they just can't go on anymore. Some of my patients going through difficult times have told me that they have thought about killing themselves. Have you had these types of thoughts?'

When beginning the assessment start with general questions before focusing on more specific details. Because the patient may minimize the severity or even the existence of suicidality it is important for the clinician to ask specific questions about the details of suicide thoughts, behaviours and plans to ensure he/she gains a clear understanding and description of these symptoms. 'Normalizing' when eliciting specific details about suicide thoughts, intent and plans can also be helpful. 'Normalizing' involves assuming that the thoughts, behaviours or plans exist:

Example
Instead of asking:

Have you made plans to kill yourself?
Ask:

What plans have you made to kill yourself?

What not to do

1 **Avoid rushing the patient or asking leading questions such as:**
   You don't have any ideas about suicide, do you?
   Such questions convey an attitude of dismissal, judgement and disinterest on the part of the clinician and may dissuade a patient who is acutely suicidal from disclosing their thoughts and intention.

2 **Do not 'interrogate' the patient or force the patient to defend his or her actions: For example, do not say:**
   Why would you do such a thing?
   Why would you even consider suicide?
   What is wrong with you?
   What is so bad in your life?

3 **Do not minimize the patient's distress. For example, do not say:**
   Oh, you are fine.
   It's not such a big thing, is it?
   Lots of people go through these kinds of things and are fine!
   Why would you feel so badly about that?

4 **Do not undercut the seriousness of the suicidal thoughts or behaviour. For example, do not say:**
   Come on... you are not really going to do anything.
   If you really wanted to die you would be dead by now.
   You'll feel better after a good night's rest.
   Get over it... you are fine.

5 **Do not avoid asking directly about suicidality even if you think the responses would be negative:**
   Be sensitive and nonjudgemental in your approach but don't avoid directly asking about suicide. If you don't ask you won't know.
   Ask: *Have you been thinking about killing yourself?*

Remember

If the patient has been having thoughts about death, feelings of hopelessness, or thoughts about suicide, addressing these issues openly in a calm, nonjudgemental, empathic manner can be a great relief. Creating an opportunity for open dialogue also creates opportunity for discovering new alternatives and choosing differently.

Acquiring collateral information

Patients may deny the presence or degree of suicidality in the clinical situation, particularly in the acute care setting or when dealing with clinicians they do not know. It is therefore essential that collateral information be obtained from individuals who are well acquainted with the patient. Family members, friends, health professionals, teachers, staff or clergy may be valuable resources for the clinician performing the assessment. These individuals can provide essential information that may influence the clinician's determination of patient risk and also provide the clinician with an understanding of the patient's existing or potential network of support. Remember that many people who die by suicide communicate their intent to others within six months of the attempt. Informants can provide important information about recent and past suicidal thoughts or plans as well as the patient's psychosocial history, current life circumstances, psychiatric and medical history, past self-injurious behaviours or suicide attempts, family environment, family history of suicide or mental illness, personality strengths and vulnerabilities, and ability to use coping strategies and mobilize external supports during times of stress.

Question

What if the patient does not directly answer questions about suicide and I think they are at risk but there is no one available to provide reliable collateral information?

Answer

Some people who are suicidal will not openly disclose suicidal ideation, intent or plans. In these situations collateral information is especially important, as described above. If collateral information is not available the clinician must rely more heavily on clinical judgement based on apparent risks, possible 'warning signs' and subjective impression. Even if suicidality is denied the clinician should look for verbal and nonverbal cues that may indicate hidden suicidal ideation, intent or plans.

1 Identifying triggers for suicidality

There is often a 'trigger' – a stressor or precipitating event – linked to suicide behaviours. Negative life events, crises or psychosocial stressors can overwhelm a person's capacity to cope. Understanding what was going on in the patient's life – the circumstances, events, thoughts feelings, and behaviours – leading up to and immediately preceding a suicide attempt can help both the clinician and the patient identify 'triggers' that elicit suicidal thoughts, feelings and behaviours.

Examples of triggers include:
- experience of trauma, victimization, abuse, bullying
- bereavement
- real/threatened or perceived loss of social support or valued/desired attachments (friends, family, partner)
- loss of identity/meaning/purpose
- loss of independence/autonomy or function (health problems)
- acute psychiatric symptoms (psychosis, depression, anxiety, panic)
- loss of hope or sense of failure
- anniversary of a significant interpersonal loss
- acute disappointments
- real/threatened or perceived embarrassment, humiliation
- real/threatened loss of job, financial security, status
- chronic health problems particularly those associated with pain, deterioration, stigmatization, cognitive impairment, dependency (males), debilitation, or burdensomeness.

2 Assessing suicide ideation

Suicide ideation refers to thoughts, fantasies, ruminations and preoccupations about death, self-harm and self-inflicted death. Active suicide ideation confers greater risk than passive suicide ideation. The greater the magnitude and persistence of the suicide thoughts, the higher the risk for eventual suicide.

In order to determine the nature and potential lethality of the patient's suicide thoughts, it is necessary to elicit the intensity, frequency, duration and persistence of the thoughts. Even if the patient initially denies thoughts of death or suicide, the clinician should ask additional questions if she or he feels the patient is not being forthcoming or is at high risk. Asking patients how they feel about the future or if they have been making or anticipating future plans may provide useful insights. Patients who are considering suicide may be ambivalent or fatalistic about the future, may describe a future devoid of hope, may express despair about the future or may not think about the future at all.

Remember that asking patients about suicide thoughts does not plant or nurture these thoughts or wishes in the patient's mind. Rather, patients often feel relieved that they have finally been given 'permission' to talk about these thoughts and feelings. Many patients who have suicide ideation feel burdened, ashamed and sinful for having such thoughts. Some are frightened by them. Some interpret these thoughts as reinforcements for their own perceived worthlessness. Opening the door to open dialogue about such thoughts and fears offers patients the opportunity to be heard and to feel understood, and can help to alleviate patients' psychological and emotional stress.

Question

How do you ask about suicide ideation?

Answer

In assessing suicide ideation it is important to ask about the presence, frequency, intensity and duration of suicide thoughts.

Remember: start general, then become more specific, but in the end always ask directly!

- 'Do you ever feel that life is not worth living?'
- 'Do you ever have thoughts about not wanting to live anymore?'
- 'Do you ever wish you were dead?'
- 'Is your death something that you have thought about recently?'
- 'Do you ever think about ending your life?'
- 'Have you had thoughts about suicide?'
- 'Have you been thinking about killing yourself?'
- 'How often do you think about killing yourself? Every day?'

- 'How long do these thoughts last when you have them? A few minutes? Hours? All day?'
- 'Are you able to manage or control these thoughts?'
- 'Do you think that you will act on these thoughts?'

3 Assessing suicide intent

Suicide intent refers to the patient's expectation of and commitment to dying by suicide. The strength of the patient's intent to die may be reflected in the patient's subjective belief in the lethality of the chosen method, which may be more relevant than the chosen method's objective lethality.

The patient's expectations and beliefs regarding the lethality of the chosen method for suicide are important to consider when estimating strength of intent. Even though the objective risk of a chosen method may be minimal, a patient's subjective conviction of the method's lethality places that patient at higher risk. The greater and clearer the suicide intent, the higher the risk for suicide.

Question

How do you ask about suicidal intent?

Answer

If someone has expressed suicide ideation, ask direct and specific questions about suicide intent. To understand 'intent' it is important to ask about the patient's expectation and commitment to die.

- 'Have you felt that you or others would be better off if you were dead?'
- 'Do you feel that life is not worth living?'
- 'Do you wish that you were dead?'
- 'If you were alone right now, would you try to kill yourself? What about in the near future?'
- 'How strongly do you want to end your life?'

4 Assessing suicide plans

The clinician must attempt to elicit the presence or absence of a suicide plan, including when, where and how a patient intends to die by suicide. This information will help inform the clinician of the potential lethality of the plan and the possibility of its success. More detailed plans are generally associated with a greater suicide risk. The lethality of the chosen method, the patient's knowledge and skill regarding the method, the absence of intervening persons or protective circumstances, the patient's preparedness to carry out the plan, the patient's access to lethal means and the patient's commitment to die by suicide all must be considered when assessing suicidal plans.

Important aspects of a suicide plan that are suggestive of the plan's potential lethality include the following:
- the chosen method
- the availability of means
- the patient's belief about the lethality of the method
- the chance of rescue
- the steps taken to enact the plan
- the patient's preparedness for death.

Patients with higher degrees of suicide intent, or more detailed and specific suicide plans, particularly those involving violent and irreversible methods, have a higher level of risk. If the patient has access to a firearm, or other lethal means, attempts should be made to ensure that these means are no longer available to the patient. Family members or other informants should be counselled to restrict access to, secure or remove these means from the patient's environment.

Question

How do you ask about suicide plans?

Answer

If someone has expressed suicide ideation, ask direct and specific questions about suicide plans, including methods, availability, belief in lethality, chance of rescue and preparations made for suicide.

- 'Have you had specific thoughts about how you might take your own life?'
- 'What have you thought about as a way to take your life?'
- 'What other things have you considered?'
- 'Have you set a time or date or place for taking your own life?'
- 'Have you obtained or do you have access to...
    o pills?
    o poison?
    o medication?
    o weapons?'
- 'Have you chosen...
    o a place to hang yourself?
    o a place to jump?
    o another method that we have not discussed?'

5. Assessing motivations for suicide

Thoughts of suicide and actions taken to end one's life are driven by feelings, beliefs, meaning or motivations that are unique to each individual and can only be understood from within that individual's context and life experience. Understanding what the 'meaning' or 'motivation' for suicide is for an individual can provide the clinician and the patient with insight into, and understanding of, the patients thoughts and feelings about themselves, their lives, their relationships, their circumstances and their future. It can also identify potential areas for intervention.

Motivation for suicide may include:
- revenge
- escape
- relief
- reunion with a dead loved one
- guilt
- self-reproach
- control
- power

6 Assessing suicide buffers

Many people have thoughts of suicide at some point in their lives – particularly during periods of severe stress. Fewer people contemplate acting on these thoughts and fewer still ever do. Thus, most people abort the 'suicide process' without any external intervention. The reasons for not acting on suicidal thoughts or carrying out suicidal plans and the internal resources used to 'stay safe' are important factors to consider when evaluating overall suicide risk.

Look for reasons for living and internal strengths for managing risk:
- 'What's important to you in your life?'
- 'What do you feel connected to? Faith? Family? Community?'
- 'What keeps you going?'
- 'Do you have a sense of purpose or meaning?'
- 'How do you manage stress?'
- 'What do you do to take care of yourself?'
- 'What has kept you from killing yourself?'
- 'What do you do that helps you deal with thoughts of suicide?'
- 'How do you manage to stay safe?'
- 'What would keep you from killing yourself now?'

Step IV Evaluating past suicide behaviours

Past suicide behaviour, including history of suicide attempts, aborted attempts or other self-harming behaviour, is a significant risk factor for suicide. When assessing a patient who has a history of a previous suicide attempt or self-injurious behaviour it is important to obtain as much detail as possible about the number of past suicide behaviours; the timing, intent, method and consequences of such behaviours; the life context in which they occurred; whether they occurred in association with intoxication or chronic use of alcohol or other substances; and the patient's current feelings about the behaviours.

Question

How do you assess past suicide behaviours?

Answer

In evaluating past suicide behaviours assess the following areas:
1 types of past suicide behaviours
2 frequency of past suicide behaviours
3 triggers of past suicide behaviours
4 lethality of past suicide behaviours
5 buffers of past suicide behaviours.

1 Types of past suicide behaviours

Remember that there are many variants of past suicide behavior, therefore inquiry into past suicide behaviours must include questions about past attempts for which help was sought or which came to the attention of health professionals, past attempts that have remained hidden, failed attempts, aborted attempts (during which the patient changed his or her mind), manipulative gestures, and other self-harm or self-injurious behaviours:

Variants of past suicide behaviour include:
- previous detected suicide attempts
- previous undetected suicide attempts
- aborted suicide attempts
- self-harming behaviours

2 Frequency of past suicide behaviours

The more frequent the attempts, the higher the risk for completed suicide, even if the lethality of the events has been low or moderate (e.g. superficial cutting, minor overdoses, etc.). In addition to enquiring about the number of past behaviours, it is important to note any change in the frequency of behaviours. If the frequency and intensity of the behaviours has been escalating, the person may be at greater risk of completed suicide.

3 Triggers of past suicide behaviours

Identifying triggers for past suicide behaviours can help the clinician and patient understand what situations or circumstances in the future might place the patient at risk for suicide; aid the clinician in targeting interventions to help the patient develop skills to manage and mitigate future risk; help build patient awareness of triggers that increase suicide risk; and help the clinician anticipate potential future periods of high risk when more frequent inquiry into suicidality may be warranted.

4 Lethality of past suicide behaviours

Understanding 'lethality' necessitates an appreciation of the nature and severity of past suicide behaviours as well as the intent of past behaviours. Remember that one severe past suicide attempt increases the risk of subsequent success.

Nature and severity
An appreciation of the nature and severity of past attempts can be gleaned from an understanding of the context in which the behaviours occurred, the lethality of the methods chosen, and the behaviours' consequences.

Context of past suicide behaviours
Information to elicit from the patient or informant regarding the context of past suicide behaviour includes the following:

- **Circumstance**   What was going on when it happened? Was there a trigger?
- **Emotional state**   How was the patient feeling leading up to and directly preceding the event? Were they feeling hopeless, guilty, humiliated, overwhelmed, afraid, tense, panicky, angry, sad, lonely, trapped...?
- **Cognitive state**   What was the person thinking leading up to and directly preceding the event? Did they believe there was no other option?
- **Behaviour**   What was the patient doing leading up to and directly preceding the event?
- **Location**   Where did the behaviour occur? Was the patient at home? Near others? In an isolated location?

- **Timing**   When did the behaviour occur? What time of day did it happen?
- **Impairment**   Was there alcohol or drugs involved? Had the patient drunk alcohol, taken medication or used drugs before it happened? Was the patient intoxicated when it happened?
- **Planning**   Was the suicide attempt planned? How long had the patient been planning it? How detailed was the plan?
- **Impulsivity**   Was the event unplanned, reactive or impulsive?

Lethality of methods used in past suicide behaviours
Information to elicit from the patient or informant regarding the methods chosen during past suicidal behaviours includes the following:

- **Lethality of method**   Did the patient choose a high-lethality method? Use of a firearm, hanging, ingestion of poison or pesticide, jumping from a significant height, and medication or drug overdose requiring medical intervention or having serious medical consequences are all examples of very lethal means.
- **Insight into the lethality of method**   Did the patient know that the means chosen was very likely to lead to a deadly outcome? Did the patient believe that the method chosen would be lethal? If the patient took a handful of iron supplements, did he or she know that ingestion of a bottle of iron tablets could be fatal? If a method of low lethality was chosen, did the patient believe he or she would die as a consequence of the chosen method (e.g. if the patient ingested a handful of nonlethal tablets)?
- **Availability of lethal means**   Was the method chosen easily accessible to the patient? How did the patient access the method chosen?

Consequences of past suicide behaviours
Information to elicit from the patient or informant regarding the consequences of past suicidal behaviours includes the following:

- **Medical severity**   Did the event result in:
  o medical intervention in the emergency department?
  o admission to a medical ward?
  o intensive care?
  o ongoing physical health consequences?

- **Treatment consequences**   Did the event result in:
  - o admission to an inpatient psychiatric ward?
  - o referral to outpatient mental health?
  - o prescription of psychiatric medication?
- **Psychosocial consequences**   Did the event result in:
  - o job loss?
  - o loss of relationship?
  - o legal issues?
  - o other negative outcome?

Intent

Evaluation of intent entails gaining an understanding of how serious and committed the patient was to die. In other words, was the suicide attempt really an attempt by the patient to take his or her life or was it an expression of frustration or anger in which the patient did not really want to die?

The following information should be elicited from the patient or informant in order to determine the patient's intent to die:

- Planning of past behaviours:
  - o Was the event planned or detailed?
- Expectation of lethality of the chosen methods:
  - o Did the patient believe the method to be lethal?
- Chance of discovery:
  - o Did the patient choose a situation in which the chance of discovery was low?
- Persons present at the time of the behaviour:
  - o Who else was present, if anyone?
- Persons to whom the attempt was communicated:
  - o Who knew about the plan before the event, if anyone?
- How the attempt was averted:
  - o Why did death not occur?
- Ambivalence toward living:
  - o Did the patient really want to die?
- Feelings about past suicidal behaviour:
  - o Does the patient regret past suicide behaviours?
- Response to the outcome:
  - o Was the person relieved or disappointed that they did not die?

- Feelings about discovery:
  - o Is the patient relieved that he or she was discovered?
  - o Was the patient disappointed that he or she was discovered?
  - o Did the patient's attempt and subsequent discovery strengthen his or her resolve to die in the future?
- Feelings about survival:
  - o Is the patient relieved that he or she did not die?
  - o Was the patient disappointed that he or she did not die?
  - o Did the patient's attempt and subsequent failure strengthen his or her resolve to die in the future?

5 Buffers of past suicide behaviours

Exploring and understanding what has been helpful in terms of managing the onset, intensity, duration and frequency of suicidal thoughts and feelings and what has dissuaded the patient from engaging in suicide behaviours despite suicide thoughts and feelings in the past can assist the clinician in developing a treatment plan that builds on the patient's self-identified coping strategies, strengths and existing internal and external supports.

Questions to ask patients who have experienced past suicidality include the following:

- 'In the past when you have had thoughts about suicide or ending your life...
  - o what kept you from acting on these thoughts?
  - o what did you do that helped you deal with these thoughts?
  - o how did you manage to stay safe?
  - o what kept you from acting on your plan?'

Step V Evaluating suicide risk and protective factors

1 Patient demographics
2 Psychiatric history
3 Psychiatric symptoms

4 Medical history
5 Family history
6 Personal history
7 Personality
8 Protective factors.

1 Patient demographics

Look for age, gender and cultural risk factors relevant to the populations in the jurisdictions in which you work.

2 Psychiatric history

Look for current or past psychiatric diagnoses, treatments, illness courses and previous hospitalizations, as well as the presence of psychiatric comorbidity, particularly if associated with substance abuse or depressive symptoms.

3 Psychiatric symptoms

Look for psychiatric symptoms associated with greater risk of suicide – sadness/depression, hopelessness, severe anhedonia, impulsivity, anxiety/panic, shame/humiliation, command hallucinations. Conducting a careful psychiatric mental status examination to identify current psychiatric signs and symptoms is essential. As greater risk is associated with depressive, anxiety, substance abuse and psychotic disorders, particular attention should be placed on the evaluation of symptoms characterizing these syndromes.

Look for psychiatric symptoms associated with increased suicide risk:

Cognitive symptoms
- hopelessness
- poor self-esteem
- cognitive skills deficits
- poor reality-testing
- command hallucinations
- intoxication.

Affective symptoms
- depressed mood

- severe anhedonia
- severe anxiety/fear/panic
- intense anger
- intense shame and humiliation
- intense loneliness.

Behavioural symptoms
- severe insomnia
- behavioural activation
- impulsivity and poor self-control
- aggression
- akathisia
- alcohol and substance misuse

Hopelessness

One of the most significant symptoms associated with increased suicide risk is the presence of hopelessness.

Hopelessness, whether in the presence or the absence of clinical depression, raises the risk of suicide. When performing a suicide assessment interview, the presence, persistence and degree of hopelessness must be evaluated.

Individuals who experience hopelessness may feel trapped by problems that appear unsolvable, situations that appear unchangeable, or pain that appears inescapable. They are often unable to see beyond their suffering and cannot grasp the possibility of better days to come.

Question

How do you ask about hopelessness?

Answer

Suggested questions include the following:
- 'Have you been feeling as if things will not change, not get better?'
- 'Have you been feeling as if it is just not worth trying any longer?'
- 'Are you pessimistic about your future?'

- 'Have you been feeling hopeless?'
- 'Have you been feeling trapped?'
- 'Have you been feeling that there is no possible solution to your problems?'

4 Medical history

Look for physical disorders associated with chronic course, poor outcomes, chronic pain, severe insomnia, fear, shame or humiliation, and loss of function.

Characteristics of the medical history associated with higher risk:

- recent diagnoses of life-threatening illness
- presence of a chronic illness
- presence of a neurological disorder
- presence of illness associated with:
  - o severe insomnia
  - o unremitting, chronic pain
  - o functional impairment
  - o cognitive impairment
  - o loss of sight or hearing
  - o disfigurement
  - o perceived burdensomeness
  - o hopelessness regarding prognosis
  - o presence of psychiatric disorder
  - o presence of psychiatric symptoms
  - o shame and humiliation

5 Family history

Look for a history of suicide, suicide attempts or psychiatric diagnoses in the immediate and extended family.

Family history of suicide or suicide attempts, particularly in first-degree relatives, or a family history of mental illness, including substance abuse, should be elicited. The circumstances of suicide or suicide attempts in the family should be discussed, including the patient's involvement and age at the time of suicide. A history of family conflict or separation, parental legal trouble, substance use, domestic violence and physical and/or sexual abuse may also increase suicide risk.

In some cases the patient may not be aware of the family history of previous suicides or suicide attempts. In other cases the patient may be aware of the events but may be reluctant to share the information for a variety of reasons, including shame, fear of stigma or discrimination, and a need to protect the family.

Remember: Suicide is an extremely sensitive subject in any culture, and the myths, stigma, secrecy and shame surrounding suicide in families are a powerful incentive to keep information hidden.

Question

How do you ask about a family history of suicide?

Answer

Be sensitive and straightforward in your approach and reassure the patient that the information provided is confidential.

- 'Many families are affected by suicide but often it is not something that families openly talk about. Do you know if anyone in your immediate or extended family has ever died by suicide?' *If yes:*
  - o 'Can you tell me what you know about that?'
  - o 'How did it affect you personally?'
- 'Do you know if anyone in your immediate or extended family ever attempted suicide?' *If yes:*
  - o 'Can you tell me what you know about that?'
  - o 'How did it affect you personally?'

6 Personal history

Look for social connectedness; quality of interpersonal relationships; life achievements; significant losses and negative life circumstances; exposure to domestic violence, abuse or neglect; recent stressful life events; or a history of childhood abuse.

The goal of this component of the assessment is to gain an understanding of pertinent positive and negative psychosocial factors affecting the patient. Important aspects of the psychosocial history include delineation of the presence or absence of external supports available to the patient at home, at school, at work, at church or in the community; gaining an understanding of the patient's current living situation and what stressors or protective factors are currently present in that environment (e.g. whether there are young children at home, whether home is a pleasant and comfortable place for the patient, the nature of the patient's current relationships with family, friends and colleagues, the presence of domestic violence, abuse or neglect); and gaining an understanding of the patient's employment status or school functioning.

This component of the assessment also provides an opportunity for the clinician to identify both acute psychosocial crises and chronic psychosocial stressors currently affecting the patient. It is often useful to perform a quick screen of common psychosocial stressors as part of the assessment. Many patients are reluctant to disclose personal information about their lives spontaneously but may do so if specifically asked about particular areas of their lives.

Areas to explore with the patient include the following:

- Quality of social network and social supports:
  - o Does the person feel alone?
  - o Are they socially isolated/living by themselves?
  - o Does the person have a network of supportive family members, friends, colleagues?
  - o Who does the person have in their life that they can turn to and count on?
  - o Is the person linked into the community?
- Quality of interpersonal relationships:
  - o Are the person's close relationships with friends and family healthy, stable, supportive?

o Are the person's close relationship with friends and family unhealthy, unstable, conflictual, abusive?
- Quality of domestic/intimate-partner relationships:
  o Is the person in an abusive relationship with their partner, family members or others?
  o Is there any evidence of domestic violence or abuse?
- Past exposure to abuse and violence:
  o Is there a history of abuse or violence in past relationships?
  o Is there a history of childhood abuse or violence?
- Presence and severity of stressors:
  o How is the person doing in terms of their roles and responsibilities at home, work/school, community, family?
  o Does the person currently have any significant childcare, financial, legal, school or work-related problems?
  o Are there intense pressures on the person to meet community-, cultural-, familial- or gender-related roles, responsibilities or expectations?
  o Has the person recently experienced the loss or breakdown of a relationship or the death of a loved one?
  o Has the person recently experienced a severe negative life event: trauma, victimization, abuse, violence?
- Recent and past exposure to suicide:
  o Has someone close to the person ever made a suicide attempt or died by suicide?
  o How has this affected the person?
  o How has it affected others who are close to the person?
  o How do the person's peers, family, community talk about or view suicide?

7 Personality

Look for ability to tolerate emotional or psychological stress, ability to manage and regulate affect, repertoire and use of healthy coping strategies, interpersonal skills, individual personality traits and thinking styles.

Insight into potentially problematic personality traits or enduring patterns of behaviour may be gained by exploring reactions to past stressful life events (particularly past losses) with the patient or informant. Such an exploration may provide important information regarding the patient's ability to handle emotional and psychological stress, use healthy coping strategies and mobilize internal and external supports.

Areas to explore with the patient and informant in the context of past stressors include:

- coping skills
- personality traits
- past responses to stress
- ability to tolerate psychological/emotional pain
- ability to satisfy psychological/emotional needs.

8 Protective factors

Look for the presence of positive social supports, a sense of connectedness or spirituality, a sense of responsibility to family, life satisfaction, intact reality-testing, positive coping skills, positive problem-solving skills and positive interpersonal relationships.

Step VI Identifying what's going on

Understanding what's going on for an individual patient requires the clinician to have an understanding of the distal factors that may confer vulnerability for suicide and the proximal factors that are relevant to the patient's current level of suicide risk.

The clinician must try to understand two fundamental questions:

1 Why?
2 Why now?

Searching for the answers to these questions will facilitate the clinician in identifying risk factors, including emotions, thoughts, behaviours and circumstances, that may be contributing to, perpetuating and precipitating acute suicide risk.

Remember that suicide is not an event, it is a process.

The suicide process is the timespan between suicide ideation and suicide action. Understanding the nature of the suicide process, its

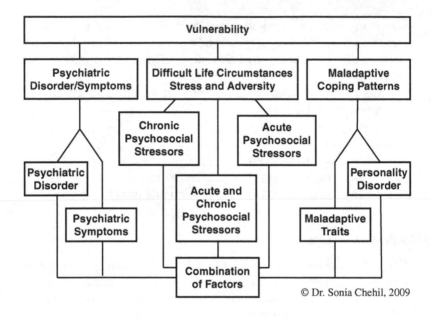

© Dr. Sonia Chehil, 2009

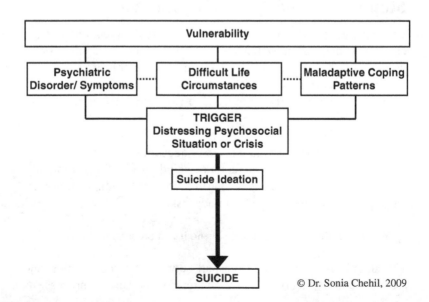

© Dr. Sonia Chehil, 2009

duration, and the modifiable factors influencing its onset and progression is essential for planning successful interventions aimed at interrupting this process and preventing the act of suicide.

Step VII Identifying targets for intervention

Some risk factors are fixed (e.g. age, gender, race/ethnicity), while others are modifiable (e.g. loss of employment, loss of housing, untreated psychiatric disorder, psychiatric symptoms, insomnia, pain associated with a chronic medical condition).

On completion of the suicide risk assessment the clinician should have a good understanding of the modifiable risk factors towards which interventions can be targeted. In addition, the clinician should have identified existing areas of strength, or protective factors that can be enhanced through appropriate intervention.

Targets for intervention include:

1 psychiatric disorders
2 psychiatric symptoms
3 chronic psychosocial stressors
4 acute psychosocial stressors
5 psychosocial crises
6 maladaptive patterns of thought, emotion and behaviour.

Remember that suicide risk assessment is both a first time of contact and a dynamic process. As a first time of contact, it is defined by a new relationship between health provider and patient. As a dynamic process, it is part of the ongoing relationship between health provider and patient (whether or not the patient has a diagnosis of a mental disorder).

Chapter 4
Putting It All Together: Tool for Assessment of Suicide Risk (TASR)

This chapter provides you with a short and succinct tool, the Tool for the Assessment of Suicide Risk, modified version (TASRm), that summarizes the information contained in Chapter 2 and 3 in a format that can be used clinically when assessing a patient for suicide risk (see Appendix A). The TASRm is divided into three sections: Individual Profile, Symptom Profile and Interview Profile. Each of these sections contains the key risk factors that must be considered when conducting a clinical evaluation of suicide risk. The TASRm does not predict suicide. It simply ensures that the clinician has obtained the minimum necessary information needed for his or her clinical assessment and is designed to complement and not replace a comprehensive clinical assessment. It can be used at the completion of the clinical interview to ensure that pertinent details necessary for the assessment of suicide risk have been addressed by the clinician. The TASRm is thus a 'bedside' tool that helps the clinician determine the 'burden of risk' for suicide.

Suicide Risk Management: A Manual for Health Professionals, Second Edition.
Sonia Chehil and Stan Kutcher.
© 2012 John Wiley & Sons, Ltd. Published 2012 by John Wiley & Sons, Ltd.

TOOL FOR ASSESSMENT OF SUICIDE RISK (TASR)

NAME: _____ Collateral: _____ Chart #: _____

INDIVIDUAL RISK PROFILE:	YES	NO
Demographic Profile: Age over 65 or between 15-35, Male > Female in most jurisdictions	☐	☐
Family History: Suicide, suicide behaviours, psychiatric disorder	☐	☐
Current/Past Psychiatric Diagnosis: Mood, Anxiety, Psychotic, Personality disorders	☐	☐
Medical Illness: Chronic, disabling, stigmatizing	☐	☐
Poor Social Supports: Living alone, isolation, exclusion, poor quality relationships	☐	☐
Alcohol/Substance Abuse	☐	☐
Domestic Problems: Domestic violence/abuse, family conflict, severe dysfunction	☐	☐
Poor Stress Tolerance: Poor Coping and Problem-Solving Skills	☐	☐
Past Suicide Behaviours: Suicide attempts, aborted attempts, self-harm	☐	☐
Abuse: Childhood or current emotional, psychological, physical, sexual abuse or violence	☐	☐

SYMPTOM RISK PROFILE:	YES	NO
Sadness/Depression/Dysphoria	☐	☐
Hopelessness	☐	☐
Severe Anhedonia	☐	☐
Severe Anxiety/Panic	☐	☐
Worthlessness/Poor Self-Esteem	☐	☐
Self-Reproach: Guilt, Self-blame, anger	☐	☐
Severe Shame/Humiliation	☐	☐
Psychosis	☐	☐
Impulsivity/Poor Self-Control	☐	☐
Anger, Violence or Aggression	☐	☐

INTERVIEW RISK PROFILE:	YES	NO
Suicide Ideation: Active: Frequency, intensity, duration **Passive:** Verbal/non-verbal cues	☐	☐
Suicide Intent: Ambivalence, degree of expectation and commitment die	☐	☐
Suicide Plan: Method, lethality, preparation	☐	☐
Past Suicide Attempt: Number, Trigger, Context, method, lethality, consequences	☐	☐
Access to Lethal Means: Availability and accessibility to lethal methods	☐	☐
Recent Alcohol/Substance Use or Intoxication	☐	☐
Suicide Trigger: Recent, evolving or anticipated psychosocial crisis/conflict/Loss	☐	☐
Unsolvable Problem: Can't see alternative solution / options	☐	☐
Intolerable State: Intense distress, despair, shame, humiliation, rejection, loneliness, pain	☐	☐
Command Hallucinations	☐	☐

RISK BUFFERS:		
Reasons For Living	☐	☐
Internal Strengths for Managing Risk	☐	☐
External Strengths for Managing Risk	☐	☐

LEVEL OF IMMEDIATE SUICIDE RISK: ☐ HIGH ☐ MODERATE ☐ LOW

Assessment Completed by: _____   DATE: _____

For each item listed, check either 'yes' (applies to the patient) or 'no' (does not apply to the patient) in the corresponding columns to the right. Then rate the overall level of suicide risk as high, moderate or low by checking the corresponding box at the bottom of the table. The rating of risk as high, moderate or low is a clinical judgement. The TASRm does not make the judgement for the clinician. The TASRm helps the clinician make her or his judgement by providing the clinician with a tool that enhances the quality of the clinical assessment.

Note: The presence of a suicide plan or high suicide intent places the patient at high risk for suicide regardless of the presence or absence of any other risk factors.

Guide to the Tool for Assessment of Suicide Risk, modified version (TASRm)

Section I Individual risk profile

This section identifies age and demographic factors as well as pertinent family, personal, medical and psychosocial history. Many people have many of these risk factors but the majority of these individuals are not suicidal. These factors only have meaning when viewed within the context of the clinical presentation. Factors within this section found to have the greatest correlation with suicide risk are listed below.

1 Demographics:
   o age and gender (males and persons between 15 and 35 years and the elderly are at highest risk in most jurisdictions), culture, socioeconomic status
2 Family History:
   o suicide, suicide behaviours, psychiatric disorder
3 Past/Present Psychiatric Diagnosis:
   o mood, anxiety, psychotic, alcohol/drug and personality disorders
4 Medical Illness:
   o chronic, disabling, stigmatizing
5 Poor Social Supports:
   o living alone, isolated, poor social network, unhealthy relationships

6 Domestic Problems:
- o violence/abuse, relationship breakdown, conflict, dysfunction
7 Poor Stress Tolerance:
- o poor self-management, coping, problem-solving, decision-making skills
8 Past Suicide Behaviours:
- o suicide attempts, aborted attempts, self-harm
9 Past/Present Abuse:
- o recent or current abuse/violence; history of childhood abuse
10 Exposure to Suicide:
- o direct (peers, family) and indirect (community, culture, social media).

Section II Symptom profile

This section addresses the current presence of psychiatric symptoms that have been associated with increased suicide risk. Again, there are many individuals who experience some or many of these symptoms but the majority of these individuals are not suicidal. These symptoms must be viewed within the context of the clinical presentation. Symptoms found to have a strong correlation with suicide risk are listed below.

1 Depression/Dysphoria
2 Hopelessness
3 Severe Anhedonia
4 Intense Emotion:
- o anxiety/panic, shame, humiliation, guilt, anger, isolation/loneliness
5 Shut Down:
- o emotional withdrawal, disengaged, noncommunicative
6 Severe Self-reproach/Worthlessness
7 Impaired Reasoning:
- o rigid thinking; poor judgement, problem-solving, decision-making
8 Poor Self-control:
- o impulsivity; poor regulation of emotions and behaviours; violence/aggression
9 Psychosis:
- o *command hallucinations
10 Problematic Alcohol/Drug Use.

Section III Interview profile

This section addresses factors identified during the interview that may place an individual at high risk of suicide whether accompanied or unaccompanied by other factors listed in Sections I and II. Overall risk is increased if risk factors from Section I are also present and overall risk is significantly increased if risk factors from Section II are also present. Items found to have the greatest correlation with suicide risk are listed below.

1 Suicide Ideation:
   o frequency, intensity, duration, persistence
2 Suicide Intent:
   o degree of ambivalence and expectation or commitment to die
3 Suicide Plan:
   o method, lethality, preparation
4 Concealed Suicidality:
   o warning signs, verbal and nonverbal cues, collateral, 'clinical intuition'
5 Past Suicide Attempt:
   o number, trigger, context, method, lethality, consequences
6 Access to Lethal Means:
   o availability of and accessibility to popular lethal methods
7 Recent Alcohol/Drug Consumption or Intoxication
8 Suicide Trigger:
   o recent, evolving or anticipated crisis/conflict/loss; victimization; trauma
9 Unsolvable Problem:
   o can't see any solution/unable or unwilling to search for alternatives
10 Intolerable State:
   o unbearable emotional, psychological, physical state or circumstance.

Section IV Risk buffers

This section addresses factors identified during the interview that may buffer suicide risk and may influence disposition and management.
1 Reasons for Living
2 Internal Strengths for Managing Risk
3 External Strengths for Managing Risk.

Section V Overall rating of risk

In this section, the clinician determines the level of suicide risk on the basis of the information obtained in the clinical interview and as identified using the TASRm items listed above. Remember that risk can be additive or exponential depending on the factors involved. The presence of a suicide plan or command hallucinations ordering suicide elevates the patient to the domain of high risk, regardless of the presence or absence of any other factors.

Level of immediate suicide risk

1 High

2 Moderate

3 Low.

Chapter 5
Special Topics in Understanding and Evaluating Suicide Risk

There are several clinical populations that deserve special address as they can present unique challenges to the clinician conducting a suicide risk assessment. This chapter will address the following:

- the chronically suicidal and the frequent, low-lethality self-harming patient
- the adolescent patient
- the elderly patient.

The chronically suicidal and the frequent, low-lethality self-harming patient

Occasionally, clinicians will encounter a patient who exhibits frequent self-harm behaviours, often of low lethality, and who may have associated affective instability and/or deficient coping and problem-solving skills. Such patients can be distressing to work with and clinicians charged with their care must learn how to appropriately assess, manage and treat these patients without allowing their own emotional responses to interfere with the quality of care provided.

Suicide Risk Management: A Manual for Health Professionals, Second Edition.
Sonia Chehil and Stan Kutcher.
© 2012 John Wiley & Sons, Ltd. Published 2012 by John Wiley & Sons, Ltd.

Examples of 'low-lethality' self-harm behaviours include the following
- Nonlethal cutting or burning of the skin.
- Nonlethal self-mutilation.
- Nonlethal overdosing on prescription or nonprescription medications, drugs or alcohol.

Other patients may be 'chronically suicidal'. That is, they may have daily thoughts of killing themselves. Although these patients may experience a waxing and waning of the intensity and persistence of these thoughts, periods of 'remission' of suicidality are often short-lived and strongly tied to psychosocial circumstances. These patients may or may not engage in self-harm behaviours.

When involved in the care of such patients, remember:
- Suicidal ideation is a risk factor for suicide.
- It is a myth that 'people who talk about it don't actually do it'.
- People with chronic suicidality and repeated low-lethality attempters do die by suicide.
- People with chronic suicidality and repeated low-lethality attempters may have an underlying treatable mental disorder.
- Chronic suicidal ideation and continued self-harm behaviours may be due to lack of response to ongoing interventions.
- Many people with chronic suicidality and many repeated low-lethality attempters may be experiencing ongoing or acute psychosocial stressors or crises that may be amenable to, or alleviated by, appropriate support and intervention.
- Each presentation requires an unbiased assessment. Situations can change and the low-lethality attempter may move to a different frame of mind in which they experience a substantive intent to die using high-lethality means. Always ask about the suicide plan.
- For the non-expert mental health clinician, these patients should be referred to specialty mental health services as soon as is possible for a comprehensive assessment.

These types of patient are challenging and will invoke ambivalent feelings in all clinicians at one time or another. It is important that clinicians be aware of their feelings about working with these patients and ensure as much as possible that these feelings do not get in the way of conducting an appropriate assessment of suicide risk. When a clinician is experiencing negative feelings towards a patient he or she may not be able to provide the careful, objective assessment of suicidality and suicide risk that is required. Remember, just because the patient has a long history of sublethal attempts does not mean that this time he or she is not serious. In all cases, a careful review and thoughtful nonjudgemental exploration is necessary.

It is not uncommon for clinicians to find themselves manipulated and emotionally entangled with such cases, and many find it very difficult to maintain clinical perspective. Clinicians may inadvertently create dependency in the patient by falling into an ongoing care-giving or rescuing role. This type of relationship is unhealthy both for the clinician, who often becomes exhausted and resentful, and for the patient, whose dependency is counter-therapeutic. If past experience with the patient or the clinician's emotional responses to the patient is interfering with the objective assessment or management of the patient, a request for a consultation should be made to another clinician.

> When feeling overwhelmed or having limited positive treatment effects – get a consultation from another clinician.

As clinicians it is our responsibility to be aware of these feelings and not to allow these feelings to interfere with clinical care. The following guidelines may be helpful:
1 Be cognizant of your own emotional, cognitive and behavioural responses to these patients.
   a Common emotional responses:
   - anger
   - hatred
   - frustration
   - disdain
   - helplessness
   - incompetence
   - anxiety
   - fear
   - resentment.

b Common cognitive responses:
- 'This person is weak.'
- 'This person is disgusting.'
- 'This person is a waste of time.'
- 'This person is just trying to get attention.'
- 'This person is taking advantage of me.'
- 'This person is manipulating me.'
- 'I wish this person would just die.'
- 'I hate this person.'
- 'I am incompetent because I cannot help this person.'
- 'This person makes me feel useless and inadequate.'
- 'If this person kills him/herself it will be my fault.'
- 'I must protect this person.'
- 'I must save this person.'

c Common behavioural responses:
- avoidance
- rejection
- overinvolvement
- overprotection
- inappropriate assumption of a 'care-taking' or 'parental' role.

2 Learn how to manage your emotional and psychological responses so that you will be able to provide a thoughtful, nonjudgemental assessment and make objective care decisions in the best interests of the patient. Obtain advice and consultation from an experienced colleague.

3 Avoid common traps:
- assumption of responsibility for the patient
- creation of dependency
- manipulation
- exploitation
- loss of personal boundaries
- enmeshment (becoming overinvolved)
- enabling
- burnout
- avoidance.

Question

What can you do?

Answer

The first step is completion of a thoughtful, nonjudgmental suicide risk assessment. This will allow you to make an informed evaluation of the patient's immediate risk for suicide. Focus on your cognitive, objective self, not your emotional, affective self.

Some of these patients may have a characterological disorder (such as borderline personality disorder) in which self-harm is a common part of the behavioural repertoire. Many more may not have a characterological disorder per se, but may have maladaptive personality traits, poor self-efficacy, poor interpersonal skills, lack of appropriate coping strategies to deal with adversity, difficulty problem-solving and seeking alternative solutions, lack of ability to manage emotional or psychological pain, and lack of ability to mobilize internal and external resources of support during times of crisis.

For patients with limited or maladaptive coping and problem-solving skills, suicidal behaviours may become an instrument for interpersonal negotiations (sometimes referred to as 'manipulative suicidality') or a means of escape when faced with difficult problems whose solutions are not immediately apparent. Use of suicidality as an overt or covert threat in order to obtain attention, medication, admission, discharge and so on from clinicians is not uncommon.

Self-harm behaviours, such as nonlethal damage to the skin (e.g. burning or cutting) and nonlethal overdosing, are very distressing to families, friends and colleagues, who often have great difficulty in understanding and managing these behaviours. Unfortunately, despite the best of intentions families, friends, and colleagues may become entangled in 'trying to keep the person safe' and thereby unwittingly become enablers of the very behaviour they wish to prevent. It is important that patients, families and care providers are able to differentiate between 'self-harm behaviour' and 'self-harm with the intention of suicide'. The caveat being that some individuals who self-harm may purposely or accidentally engage in self-injury using methods of fairly significant lethality (such as ingestion of large amounts of aspirin or acetaminophen), which may either result in death or cause significant physical damage.

In some cases, 'hidden' psychiatric disorders such as mood, anxiety or substance-use disorders may be present. Psychiatric symptoms, such as hopelessness in depression or auditory hallucinations in psychosis, may underlie chronic suicidality. For patients not receiving treatment, initiation of appropriate treatment for the underlying symptoms by either psychotherapy (such as cognitive behaviour therapy for hopelessness) or medications (such as antipsychotics for schizophrenia) may ameliorate the suicidality. For patients receiving treatment a reevaluation of current and past treatments, treatment efficacy, treatment compliance and treatment side effects is warranted, and lack of response or partial response to ongoing interventions should be addressed by optimizing or changing current treatment modalities.

The results of the consultation should be openly discussed with the patient and others. Impressions regarding diagnosis and decisions on management and intervention must be unambiguous and clearly communicated to the patient, the patient's family and all members of the health care team, including those who may have intermittent contact with the patient in the community or the accident and emergency department, and must be documented in the patient's records.

The use of the lethality criteria in the TASRm can help guide clinical decision-making. If the clinician is not certain about the degree of the patient's risk then she or he may find it reasonable to provide for a short period of safe observation (ranging from a few hours to one day) during which the patient's risk for suicide may become more clear.

Question

Why do individuals engage in self-harm behaviours?

Answer

The reasons are diverse and vary from one individual to another. Some patients describe feeling 'numb' or gaining a 'sense of relief' from psychological and emotional pain during and after self-inflicted physical pain or injury. Others report a brief feeling of euphoria associated with self-harm behaviours such as cutting. Some report using self-harm as a means of self-punishment, others as a means of decompressing anger. Some use self-harm behaviour as a means to control and manipulate others, particularly those with whom they are emotionally linked.

The adolescent patient

In Western countries, suicide is often one of the top three causes of death in young people between the ages of 15 and 24. Risk for completed suicide is highest among older youth (late teens to early twenties), and in most countries boys are more likely to die by suicide than girls, whereas girls make more suicide attempts than boys. In the USA, among 15–19 year-olds and among 20–24 year-olds the ratio of male to female suicide is estimated to be $4:1$ and $6:1$ respectively.

Stressful life events and pressures from home, school, work, peers and community are all part of the normal process of growing and accumulating new experiences and life skills, and the vast majority of young people will negotiate their teen years and early adulthood successfully (some with a few hiccups along the way) and grow to lead fulfilling and productive lives. However, some young people have greater difficulty with the transition from childhood to adulthood, and some won't make it. Suicide in young persons, like suicide in adults, is complex, with multiple dynamic interplaying factors contributing to the event in each individual case.

Psychiatric disorders most commonly associated with youth suicide include mood disorders (depression, hypomania-mania or mixed states), particularly when accompanied by alcohol- or other substance-abuse disorders, and disruptive behaviour disorders (particularly conduct disorder in boys). Depression is the strongest attributable risk factor in girls. Psychiatric symptoms associated with higher risk of suicide in youth are similar to those in adults, with hopelessness, irritability, agitation, impulsivity and aggression being particularly significant. Other factors associated with higher risk include low self-esteem, poor self-confidence and a pattern of distorted negative self-appraisal and self-blame. In addition to a history of suicidal behaviour and parental psychopathology (particularly depression and substance abuse), poor communication between the young person and his or her parents, rigid or unrealistic parental pressure or expectation, and rigid or unrealistic cultural pressure or expectation may also be important factors to consider when assessing suicide risk in teenagers.

Suicidal thoughts are relatively common amongst adolescents. Many young people will endorse contemplating 'ending their lives', particularly during or in the aftermath of a major stressor. However, very few youth will actually engage in deliberate acts of self-harm and even fewer will commit suicide. Suicidal ideation in and of itself does not indicate psychopathology or need for intervention in teenagers. In children, however, expression of suicidal ideation warrants serious attention. Young children may not appreciate the 'finality' of death and therefore may unwittingly commit suicide, not realizing that they will not come back. Suicidal behaviours, on the other hand, are more likely to be associated with psychopathology including mood and anxiety disorders, disruptive behaviour disorders and substance-use disorders. Suicidal behaviours are more common in girls than in boys and are a significant risk factor for completed suicide in both sexes.

Self-harm behaviours and completed suicide in adolescence are often preceded by a trigger (usually an acute psychosocial stressor) such as the breakup of a relationship, peer rejection, difficulties at home, or trouble at school or with the law. In general, young people are more likely than adults to be short-sighted, impulsive and exhibit immature coping strategies, particularly when under stress. It is always important to appreciate the significance of a stressor from the perspective of the individual, taking into account his or her sociocultural-religious background, experience, level of emotional maturity and psychological/cognitive sophistication. Stressors that may be of particular concern during adolescence include those associated with the following:

- experienced or perceived shame or humiliation
- experienced or perceived bullying, social exclusion or rejection
- experienced or perceived failure
- experienced or perceived fear of loss of a loved one.

Question

There are many changes that take place during adolescence; how can you tell if the changes are benign or potentially dangerous?

Answer

In young people, differentiating between 'disturbance', which may be indicative of a major underlying problem, and 'distress', which is relatively benign (a normal stress response to difficult life events and challenges), can be challenging even for the seasoned clinician. With hindsight, friends and relatives of young people who are found to be suffering from a mental disorder such as depression, substance abuse or schizophrenia will recall seeing 'warning signs' that something was not right in the months or even years before the individual accessed care and received a diagnosis. These warning signs are often attributed to normal 'growing pains' until the underlying problem reaches a severity that necessitates help-seeking.

Some of the warning signs listed below are commonly expressed at one time or another by most, if not all, adolescents. Many of these warning signs are nonspecific and ambiguous, and taken separately may be just a normal part of growing up. On the other hand, if these warning signs represent a clear change in a young person's personality, behaviour or functioning they may be signals of a serious underlying problem. For example, changes in personality, behaviour or functioning may herald the onset of a neurological or psychiatric disorder (such as a seizure disorder, mood disorder, anxiety disorder, substance-use disorder, undetected learning disability or, more rarely, schizophrenia); they may signal that the child or youth has or is experiencing a severe stressor or trauma; or they may be indicative of an underlying medical problem.

Warning signs that something may be wrong include:
- significant changes in home, school, work or social function
- significant changes in personality
- significant changes in behaviour
- withdrawal from family
- withdrawal from friends and social activities
- loss of interest in activities previously enjoyed

- neglect of personal appearance
- significant change in weight (especially weight loss when not dieting)
- sleep difficulties (especially in sleep continuity and early waking)
- persistent self-deprecating comments
- increased use of drugs and/or alcohol
- dysphoria, intense sadness or despair
- increased irritability, anger or aggression
- increased difficulty in controlling emotions
- increased risk-taking or impulsivity
- preoccupation with death or people who have died by suicide
- suicide or death as the theme of conversation, schoolwork or artwork
- hopelessness as the theme of conversation, schoolwork or artwork
- giving away valued possessions.

How do you know when to be concerned?

As in adults, understanding these risk factors will not allow you to predict with certainty who will or will not commit suicide, but it can assist clinicians in identifying young people who may be at risk for suicide, in performing a suicide risk assessment, and in determining the most appropriate level of intervention.

Family history of suicide and mental illness

As in adults, a family history of suicide or mental illness increases the risk for suicide in teenagers. Some youngsters may not be aware of this history; others may be very reluctant to share it. Obtaining this history from family members is essential. Always ask the teen and a family member (usually the mother, if available) about a family history of suicide.

Collateral history and teen suicide

Many adolescents may be very reluctant to discuss suicidal ideation, intent or plans. This reluctance can be heightened in a situation in which the adolescent feels forced to comply or participate or when they do not relate to the health professional. Thus, a standard procedure when assessing a teenager should be to obtain a collateral history from a parent or other responsible adult (such as a teacher). However, a teenager should always be offered an interview separate from parents or guardians.

Confidentiality and the teenager

An adolescent may be reluctant to discuss personal information with a clinician, particularly if the adolescent believes that he or she or his or her friends may 'get into trouble', or if the adolescent thinks that the clinician may tell their parents. Sometimes these fears may seem inconsequential to the clinician but be very important to the teenager.

As a clinical rule of thumb, it is useful to tell the teenager that information obtained in the interview will be held in confidence unless that information pertains to something that can seriously harm or injure the youth (such as risk for suicide). In such cases the responsible adult must be informed but the clinician must involve the adult in a manner that is respectful and protective of the young person.

Specific serotonin reuptake inhibitors (SSRIs) and adolescent suicide

An interest in the relationship between SSRI use and teenage suicide surfaced following a review of unpublished clinical trial data. Although some commentators (especially the media) struggled hard to forge a causal link between SSRI use and teen suicide, multiple independent investigations of the data by qualified groups and individuals showed that contrary to this perception, not only was SSRI use not associated with completed suicide but it was possibly a significant factor in treating teen depression and decreasing teen suicide. Ecological data have demonstrated that jurisdictions with high antidepressant prescription rates for young people are characterized by lower rates of youth suicide. In the USA and Canada, a decrease in SSRI prescriptions following the FDA 'black box' warning has been paralleled with increases in youth suicide rates.

SSRI use, however, can be associated with increased suicidal ideation and self-harm or suicidal behaviours in some teens. These medications should only be used by qualified health professionals with careful monitoring and proper patient/parent education. Different national professional bodies/authorities have different recommendations regarding the use of SSRIs in young people (for example NICE in the UK, AACAP in the USA, CACAP in Canada). If these are available in your jurisdiction it is a good idea to use them to guide your practice.

The Kutcher Adolescent Depression Scale (KADS)

Many of the self-rated instruments often used to measure depression in adolescents (12–18 years) have limited or unknown reliability, validity and sensitivity to change over time in this age group. This is unfortunate because self-report scales have the potential to provide useful information quickly and cheaply. In view of the need for a quickly administered, valid, sensitive-to-change depression-rating scale for adolescents, one of the authors (S.K.) has devised a self-report scale: the Kutcher Adolescent Depression Scale (KADS). The KADS is a validated tool that can identify teens who have depression and who may be suicidal. The original version of the KADS contained 16 items. The scale provided and described in this manual is the 6-item KADS.

The 6-item version of KADS was developed as a screening tool for depression in youth. This scale can be completed and hand-scored quickly and easily and is ideal for screening and interview purposes in clinical settings.

The 6-item version of the KADS is reproduced in Appendix B. It is also available in numerous different languages free of charge at www.teenmentalhealth.org. An adolescent version of the TASR, the TASR(A), can also be found in different languages free of charge at the same Web site.

Other youth self-report depression screening instruments are available. These include the Beck Scale and the Reynolds Scale. They can be found through any of the Web search engines (such as Google).

The elderly patient

In most developed countries the highest rates of suicide are seen in the elderly, particularly among males. Although proportionally suicide is not as common a cause of death in the elderly as in younger age groups, this does not mean that suicide in the elderly is not a concern – quite the contrary. In many Western countries, the age cohort demonstrating the greatest proportional growth is the elderly, and with the baby-boom bulge now reaching this demographic, clinicians can expect to encounter more situations in which they will be called upon to assess an elderly patient for suicide risk.

There are a number of factors that may contribute to the higher risk of completed suicide in the elderly. In general, the elderly are less physically resilient, are more likely to be suffering from a variety of physical illnesses and are more likely to have access to medication that taken in excess or in combination has a greater likelihood of lethality. In many societies the elderly are more likely to be living alone and to be more socially isolated than their younger counterparts, and are therefore less likely to disclose suicidality and less likely to be discovered or rescued following a suicide attempt. The elderly are also more likely to live in poverty; are more likely to be dependent on others; are more likely to have experienced losses related to life transitions, retirement and loss of functional abilities; and are more likely to have suffered numerous personal losses and to have experienced profound grief resulting from the death of a spouse, close friends and family members. In addition, the elderly are more likely to face uncertainty, ambivalence and anxieties about their future. The elderly are also vulnerable to being victims of violence, abuse and neglect.

In addition, the elderly are less likely to engage in impulsive suicidal behaviours and are more likely to have reached a definitive decision about ending their life by suicide after much contemplation and planning. Elders who commit suicide generally demonstrate a greater determination to die than younger individuals, as evidenced by the fact that suicidal elders give fewer warnings signs of their ideas and plans, use more violent and potentially lethal methods to commit suicide, and engage in suicidal behaviours that involve greater planning and resolve.

Another important issue that is too often overlooked in the elderly is major depressive disorder, or clinical depression. Many people, including health professionals, believe that thoughts about suicide or ruminations about death are normal in the elderly and dismiss depression as a normal part of ageing. This is a myth. Most people feel quite satisfied with their lives as they grow older. When depression occurs it can cause significant suffering to the elderly person and can lead to the worsening of any underlying medical conditions that they may have. In addition, depression in an elderly person may be due to side effects of medications used to treat health conditions or may be caused by an underlying medical illness. Depressive episodes in the elderly tend to be more severe, more frequent and carry a greater risk of chronicity than episodes occurring in younger adults. Depression in the elderly is probably more common than once thought, particularly for patients who are medically ill or residing in nursing home facilities. Loss of a spouse, friends and family members, as well as loss of health and the burden of resulting disabilities, are frequent stressors faced by the elderly that may increase their vulnerability to developing depression. Further, depression in the elderly significantly increases suicide risk, particularly for those who experience extended episodes that are inadequately treated. Unfortunately, depression in the elderly often goes unrecognized and untreated.

Elderly patients with depression are less likely than younger individuals to experience depression as sadness or low mood. Rather, they may complain of 'not feeling like themselves', or of feeling useless, dissatisfied and disinterested in things around them. Elderly individuals who are depressed may appear more irritable, fretful or agitated. They are more likely to experience mood-congruent delusions, often with prominent guilt-ridden, self-reproaching themes. The elderly are also more likely than younger individuals to experience depressive symptoms as physical problems and to attribute difficulties related to depression to medical illnesses. Physical manifestations of depression in the elderly include sleep problems, weight loss, digestive problems, constipation, muscle aches and pains, headaches, weakness, lethargy, fatigue and dizziness. All of these symptoms are vague and can be difficult to differentiate from other medical disorders or medication side effects.

In addition, the elderly tend to suffer more profound cognitive dysfunction when they are depressed compared to younger individuals. The cognitive dysfunction includes memory problems, difficulties with decision-making and difficulties with organizing and accomplishing tasks, and can be particularly difficult to differentiate from the symptoms of dementia. In fact, depression which onsets for the first time in the elderly can be a harbinger of a dementing illness, such as Alzheimer's disease, or may signal the occurrence of an ischaemic event, such as a silent stroke. This diagnostic conundrum can lead to both misdiagnosis and failure to treat late-onset depression, which can result in progressive disability for the affected individual. This is a particularly unfortunate outcome as late-onset depression is a very treatable disorder and the cognitive dysfunction which accompanies it reverses once the depression resolves.

Question

How do you differentiate late-onset depression from dementia?

Answer

Depression in the elderly is often heralded by the onset of physical problems such as changes in sleep patterns, changes in appetite, and fatigue. Cognitive problems develop acutely rather than insidiously over many months, which is more in keeping with a dementia. In addition, patients with depression generally demonstrate a rapid progression of symptoms over several weeks once the depressive episode declares itself and often there is a personal or family history of major depressive disorder.

The cognitive difficulties typical of late-onset depression tend to develop acutely rather than insidiously, as is more typical of a dementing illness, and tend to be patchy and inconsistent with patterns typically observed with the different types of dementia. In contrast to patients with dementia, who often overlook or appear unaware of their cognitive deficits, the patient with late-onset depression may overstate their impairment, offer detailed complaints of their difficulties, and make minimal efforts to respond to questions, with many 'I don't know' answers. These individuals are more likely to highlight their failures, appear self-blaming, express feelings of hopelessness and worthlessness, and have thoughts of suicide.

While the same general risk factors discussed earlier in this monograph apply equally to the elderly, the clinician should be aware of the need to assess for suicide risk at times following intimate loss and other life crises. The presence of unexplained physical symptoms such as bruising or fractures should suggest the possibility of elder abuse or substance abuse. In these circumstances, the clinician should strongly consider assessment for suicide risk.

As with teenagers, it is important to obtain collateral history. There may be memory difficulties that make communication of suicide intent problematic, or the stigma against suicide may be greater in older compared to younger people. The wish to not be a burden on family or friends may also be associated with a decreased willingness to report suicidal thoughts or plans. The appropriate assessment of suicide risk in the elderly includes a discussion about 'what's going on' with those who know the patient best.

Factors which may increase the risk of suicide in the elderly include the following:

- presence of unrecognized or inadequately treated clinical depression.
- presence of chronic medical conditions and end-of-life illnesses.
- onset of dementia.
- unrecognized substance abuse (especially alcohol).
- being single, divorced or living alone.
- high rates of intimate losses and grief: spouse, family members, close friends.
- loneliness, social isolation and limited social supports.
- loss of social role and status.
- loss of physical functionality and increased dependency on others.
- unrecognized elder abuse (by family or caregivers).
- previous suicide attempt.

Chapter 6
Suicide Prevention

Suicide-prevention strategies

There are two evidence-based approaches to suicide prevention: population-based strategies and strategies targeting high-risk groups or individuals. Building and strengthening health-system capacity to provide a continuum of evidence-informed care services for people with mental disorders, means restriction, gatekeeper training, and implementation of crisis-support programmes are examples of evidence-informed population-based strategies. In addition, programmes that focus on strengthening coping and problem-solving skills and programmes that strengthen and enhance the availability of and access to networks and systems of support are important population-based interventions. Targeted approaches include the provision of evidence-informed care and treatment for individuals experiencing a suicidal crisis, early identification and assessment of persons at risk for suicide, systems for early identification and appropriate treatment of mental disorders, and the implementation of targeted interventions for modifiable risk factors.

Although many universal and targeted interventions for suicide prevention have been implemented in countries and communities around the world, few have been empirically studied and evaluated in either developing or developed countries. Of those that have been evaluated, few have been shown to impact suicide rates. To date, the most promising evidence-based interventions include health-provider education, means restriction and gatekeeper training.

Suicide Risk Management: A Manual for Health Professionals, Second Edition.
Sonia Chehil and Stan Kutcher.
© 2012 John Wiley & Sons, Ltd. Published 2012 by John Wiley & Sons, Ltd.

Population issues in suicide prevention

The association between mental disorders – particularly depression and alcohol and other substance abuse – and suicide globally is clear and interventions that promote the early identification of and appropriate, effective and continuous treatment for mental disorders by health providers have been demonstrated to be the most effective method for the prevention of suicide. Gatekeeper training has also been demonstrated to be an empirically supported suicide-prevention approach and has been implemented and studied in many different populations, including military personnel, school personnel, peer helpers and clinicians. Gatekeeper training as an intervention focuses on helping specific groups of people identify individuals at high risk for suicide and then refer them for assessment, care or support to the most appropriate available service. The caveat here of course is that the effectiveness of health-provider and gatekeeper training as suicide-prevention strategies relies on systems being in place to support the provision of accessible and effective mental health care (both in specialty mental health services and in primary care).

The restriction of community access to highly lethal means has also been demonstrated to be an effective suicide-prevention strategy. The suicide method chosen is a significant factor in determining risk of death by suicide. Availability and acceptability of methods for suicide vary across regions, nations, cultures and communities. Ease of access to specific means and cultural awareness, attitudes and beliefs associated with different means are believed to influence the choice of method used in different communities and cultures. Successful examples of means restrictions, whether from planned intervention or secondary to national or local policy change, include the detoxification of domestic gas, the introduction of catalytic converters in vehicles, passage of firearm-control laws, modification of drug packaging, installation of barriers at jump sites, restrictions on the availability of barbiturates, and regulation and control of toxic pesticides and herbicides.

Globally, the most common methods of suicide are ingestion of pesticides, the use of firearms, and medication overdose. In developing countries, particularly in rural areas, ingestion of pesticides is the main method of suicide. An estimated 30% of global suicide deaths are believed to involve ingestion of pesticide. Although reliable data on suicide attempts in developing countries are scarce, the gender disparity in suicide behaviour that is so striking in developed countries is less dramatic in developing countries. This may partially be accounted for by the high case fatality associated with pesticide ingestion. Where pesticide poisoning is the most common method of choice, survival following an attempt is unlikely.

Most pesticide-related deaths are believed to be impulsive acts of self-harm. In Asia, for example, most cases of pesticide suicides are believed to be unplanned, impulsive actions in response to crisis situations or stressful life events, and not highly correlated with mental disorder. Rather, impulsive suicide deaths in these countries are highly correlated with the availability and ease of access to toxic pesticides. Pesticides used by victims are often highly accessible – often found within or near the homes of the victim. In contrast to the relative low toxicity of common substances used in suicide attempts in the west, case fatality following ingestion of commonly used pesticides – paraquat and aluminum phosphide – is estimated to be over 70%. Further, the window for successful intervention in pesticide poisoning is very short and in many developed countries lack of access to and availability of appropriate medical care services, antidotes to pesticide poisoning, and properly trained health professionals to manage pesticide poisoning is a significant barrier to potential life-saving treatments. Given this startling information, local and national policy decisions and community interventions that promote the restriction of access to and the availability of pesticides, mandate the safe storage of pesticides, and promote improved access to and availability of professionals appropriately trained to treat pesticide poisonings may dramatically reduce suicide rates globally.

A number of interventions popularly considered to be very effective in reducing suicide rates, including suicide telephone hotlines and school-based suicide-education programmes, have shown little or no substantial positive effect on decreasing suicide rates. The table below outlines the usefulness of a number of suicide-intervention programmes for youth. The effect of national suicide-prevention programmes when mental health treatment variables are controlled for is not clear.

Usefulness of suicide-intervention programmes for youth

No demonstrated benefit	Possibly harmful	Harmful	Likely benefit	Definite benefit
Suicide hotlines School-based peer-counselling programmes	School suicide-awareness programmes Focus groups or special school lectures on suicide Suicide screening in schools	Sensational media coverage of suicides	School mental health literacy programmes – when linked with good access to mental health care Restricted access to firearms and other available lethal means Increasing and enforcing legal drinking age	Early identification and treatment of mental disorders – the use of 'gatekeeper' programmes and primary-care physician training Early identification and effective treatment of young people with suicide risk factors and warning signs Timely suicide risk assessment and focused intervention by health professionals

In some jurisdictions community suicide awareness and other universal 'prevention' programmes are popular and commercially available 'suicide-prevention' programmes are frequently promoted. The evidence that these expensive and broad-based applications are more effective in preventing suicide than targeted interventions that improve suicide risk identification, evaluation and interventions by gatekeepers and health providers is to our knowledge not clear. Research into suicide prevention is progressing at a rapid rate and strategies currently under investigation may better help our understanding of what works and what does not work at the population level and inform community-based applications in the future.

Individual issues in suicide prevention

For the individual, suicide-prevention methods should include early identification and appropriate treatment of mental disorders, recognition of warning signs of suicide risk, early identification and assessment of persons at risk for suicide, appropriate acute safety management for suicidal patients, and the implementation of targeted interventions for modifiable risk factors.

Chapter 7
Suicide Intervention

All patients identified as having warning signs of or being at risk for suicide must have a comprehensive suicide assessment performed. The information obtained from the suicide risk assessment will inform clinical decision-making regarding the patient's immediate, short-term and longer-term care needs. Use of the Tool for the Assessment of Suicide Risk (TASR) (see Chapter 4 and Appendix A) can assist clinicians in determining the level of suicide risk.

On completion of the suicide risk assessment the clinician should be able to make an informed clinical judgement regarding the patient's level of suicide risk and the level of care required. In addition, the clinician should have a good understanding of what the modifiable risk factors are towards which interventions can be targeted, as well as existing areas of strength or protective factors that can be enhanced through appropriate intervention.

Step 1: Address the immediate safety of the patient

Any patient presenting with risk factors or warning signs for suicide should not be left alone or unattended and any potentially dangerous objects should be removed from the patient's environment. All patients at risk must be asked if they have recently done anything to harm or attempt to kill themselves and if they have anything with them that they are planning to use to harm or kill themselves. If the

Suicide Risk Management: A Manual for Health Professionals, Second Edition.
Sonia Chehil and Stan Kutcher.
© 2012 John Wiley & Sons, Ltd. Published 2012 by John Wiley & Sons, Ltd.

patient has anything on their person that could be used to harm or kill themselves – a weapon, razor blade, medication, poison, etc. – these items must be immediately removed from the patient's possession. Any patient presenting with a suicide in process requires immediate medical assessment and intervention.

For patients who present in acute psychosocial crisis the basic principles of crisis management should be instituted as part of the risk assessment:

1 Ensure the physical safety of the patient, as outlined above.
2 Defuse emotional stress by allowing ventilation of feelings.
3 Allow the patient to tell his/her story and help him/her understand their situation and reactions.
4 Provide practical support and reassurance.
5 Help the patient identify coping strategies and skills used to get through difficult times in the past.
6 Help the patient problem-solve and identify alternative solutions and ways of coping.
7 Mobilize supportive family and friends to assist in providing support, problem-solving and understanding.
8 Help connect the patient to available supports, services and resources in their community.

The focus of crisis management is to ensure the patient's immediate safety and to defuse severe emotional distress. If the patient is unable to gain emotional control or is unable to think rationally and is overtly or covertly expressing suicidality, they should be considered high-risk until proven otherwise.

Step 2: Determine required level of care

Not all patients who are determined to be at risk for suicide require admission to hospital or another care facility. In some settings, admission to an acute care or crisis facility may be the most appropriate choice – if such services are accessible and available. In another setting, care may be effectively and appropriately provided on an outpatient basis. The determination of level of care is based on level of risk as well as on the types of crisis care service and support available and accessible to the individuals and their family in their community, and the availability of strong primary social supports.

For patients deemed to be at high and imminent risk of suicide, their protection is of paramount concern. For such patients, treatment in a secure and protected environment such as an inpatient or crisis bed is often necessary as outpatient and community services may not be sufficient to provide the level of intensive support required. Admission to a secure inpatient setting may be voluntary or involuntary. As far as possible, admission to an inpatient setting should occur with the patient's consent and in collaboration with primary social supports. If a patient who is judged to be at imminent risk of suicide refuses admission to a secure facility, involuntary commitment must be considered and may be necessary. All clinicians must be aware of the legal requirements regarding involuntary commitment in the jurisdiction in which they practise. In some cases, patients deemed to be at risk for suicide may be safely and effectively treated as outpatients if there are capable family members and others available to provide around-the-clock support and supervision and to whom the responsibility of oversight can be entrusted.

Step 3: Acute safety planning in hospital or at home

If an acutely suicidal patient is hospitalized, the clinicians must ensure that the hospital staff is fully aware of the patient's suicide risk and that the necessary precautions are taken to ensure patient safety. For example, the patient should not have access to means of self-harm (such as a belt that can be used for hanging, scissors that can be used for cutting, freedom of movement that can lead to jumping from a height). Patients who are highly suicidal may require constant or frequent observation and monitoring by responsible staff. The patient's level of suicide risk should be reviewed at least daily and decisions regarding freedom of movement and activity level (access to the general ward, interaction with other patients, participation in ward activities, off-unit privileges) should be reviewed and adapted based on repeated risk assessment.

If a patient is to be discharged in the care of their family or other supports, patient safety takes precedence over patient confidentiality and the clinician must develop a collaborative safety plan involving the patient and the patient's caregivers that outlines actions to be taken to ensure the home environment is safe and what to do if the patient's condition deteriorates. Caregivers should be provided with education regarding suicide in general and suicide risk and protective factors relevant to the patient, and should also be involved in decisions about hospitalization and in recommendations for immediate and long-term treatment. Caregivers should be advised to remove potential risks such as medications, weapons, sharps and other potential means of self-harm from the patient's environment. Work with the patient and caregivers to develop a safety plan that includes coping strategies to defuse or manage intense emotional or psychological pain, strategies to manage suicidal thoughts, lists of useful contact numbers of services and supports available in the community and instructions on when and how to seek professional help. It is advised that the patient and caregivers be instructed to seek assistance immediately if there is an increase in suicidality or if the caregivers or patient do not feel able to cope and ensure safety at home. In addition, the clinician should ensure that specific arrangements for reassessment and follow-up within 12–24 hours of discharge are made before the patient leaves the clinic or hospital. The intensity of ongoing support and supervision, and the frequency of follow-up and monitoring of risk, will depend on the patient's level of suicide risk.

Whether the patient is admitted to an inpatient facility or is discharged home with outpatient follow-up, the clinician must always make a detailed note in the patient's chart explaining his or her action, the level of suicide risk based on objective and subjective data, identified risk and protective factors contributing to, precipitating and maintaining risk, details of any treatment or interventions made, and the components of the safety management plan.

Question

What if a proper suicide assessment cannot be performed?

Answer

If a clinician is unable to complete an assessment or if he or she feels unsure of the patient's safety following completion of the assessment (even if the patient adamantly denies suicide risk) it is reasonable to admit the patient to a care facility and reassess in 8–12 hours. Suicidal patients who are intoxicated and are therefore unable to cooperate with an assessment should be held for observation until they have detoxified and a proper mental status examination can be carried out. In no case should a suicidal intoxicated patient be allowed to leave the clinic or hospital alone or in the company of anyone else.

Question

What about the suicide-prevention contract?

Answer

The suicide-prevention contract is sometimes used by clinicians in emergency rooms as well as acute and long-term inpatient and community settings. The success of the suicide-prevention contract (sometimes referred to as the 'no-harm' contract) is probably attributable to the strength of the therapeutic relationship between the patient and the clinician with whom the contract is formed. By itself, the no-harm contract has not been shown to be an effective preventive measure. In fact, it may give clinicians a false sense of security that may impair their ability objectively to assess suicide risk and may affect their judgement in terms of formulating treatment plans. The no-harm contract is not a substitute for a proper clinical assessment. It is our opinion that it has limited value in suicide prevention and generally should not be used. When all is said and done, the assessment and treatment of suicide risk relies on informed clinical judgement, not on a clinician–patient contract.

Step 4: Identify areas for intervention

Once the patient's immediate safety is attended to, precipitating triggers as well as any identified modifiable physical, emotional, cognitive, behavioural and psychosocial risk factors contributing to the patient's suicidality will need to be addressed. Treatment and intervention should be instituted to reduce current and future suicide risk and include both biological and psychosocial interventions.

Targets for intervention include:
1 psychosocial crisis
2 psychiatric disorders
3 psychiatric symptoms
4 psychosocial stressors
5 acute psychosocial stressors
6 maladaptive patterns of thought, emotion and behaviour.

Appropriate pharmacological and psychosocial treatment of an existing psychiatric disorder and psychiatric symptoms can significantly reduce suicide risk. If a patient is found to have an untreated psychiatric disorder, appropriate treatment should be initiated. For patients already receiving treatment for a diagnosed psychiatric condition, treatment should be optimized following review of past and current treatment, treatment responses, treatment compliance and treatment side effects.

Cognitive behavioural techniques have demonstrated efficacy in reducing suicidal ideation and improving self-esteem, hopelessness and impulsivity across a variety of disorders. Pharmacological interventions that have been demonstrated to specifically reduce suicidality include the appropriate treatment of antidepressants – particularly the newer and safer SSRIs – in clinical depression, the use of clozapine in patients with psychosis and the use of lithium in mood disorders. The long-term effectiveness of lithium therapy in reducing suicide in bipolar patients is well established. Patients who are being treated with lithium and who discontinue that medication quickly may be at higher suicide risk.

For individuals in crisis, provision of therapeutic support and/or temporary respite can allow time and space to recover coping strategies, gain perspective and see options beyond suicide. Once the acute crisis response has settled, work with the patient and primary social supports to develop a preventive strategy focused on reducing the likelihood of a future suicide crisis:
- Review the circumstances leading up to the suicide crisis.
- Identify specific triggers, emotions, thoughts and behaviours that contributed to the crisis response.
- Review the patient's internal strengths and any coping strategies successfully used in the past.
- Review the patient's availability and use of external supports.

- Use brief supportive and problem-focused interventions to reinforce and expand existing internal and external strengths and to develop areas of identified weakness.
- Make use of brief supportive and problem-focused interventions to:
  o improve stress management
  o strengthen adaptive coping and problem-solving skills
  o encourage self-care: healthy diet, regular exercise, good sleep hygiene
  o discourage alcohol and substance use
  o manage and control maladaptive thoughts, including suicide ideation, hopelessness and self-reproach
  o manage and control intense negative emotions
  o develop strategies to improve impulsivity and behavioural control
  o expand the patient's social support network.
- Connect the patient with available community supports and services.

The same strategies outlined above can be used to address acute and chronic psychosocial stressors believed to contribute to suicide risk.

For patients with inadequate or maladaptive coping strategies, psychotherapeutic interventions that focus on skill-building and problem-solving, such as cognitive behavioural therapy, can be very helpful. Dialectic behaviour therapy has been demonstrated to decrease suicide attempts in personality-disorder patients in some studies.

Step 5: Provide ongoing monitoring and evaluation

Suicidality is not an illness, it is a symptom of an underlying problem. Interventions for suicidality are aimed at reducing immediate and future suicide risk by managing underlying risk factors and enhancing protective factors. A safety plan, such as the one provided in Appendix C, should be developed for all patients at risk for suicide and suicide behaviours. Ongoing monitoring and risk assessment is essential and should reflect the level of suicide risk for a given patient. Continuing therapeutic contact over the long term may be particularly important in decreasing suicide rates in individuals with psychiatric disorders.

There is no 'cookbook recipe' that can be followed to treat the suicidal patient. It is the application of the above basic principles to the individual case that matters. In each case the clinician must determine the relative risk of suicide. The use of the TASR in this risk assessment can help the clinician complete a thorough risk assessment.

The cases studies in Chapter 10 allow the clinician, individually or as part of a self-study group, to practise application of the TASR. The authors recommend that, following a reading of this monograph, the clinician immediately practise the application of the TASR to at least two or three different cases so as to enhance learning of this material by its application.

Chapter 8
Post-suicide Intervention: Caring for Survivors

Sometimes, despite our best interventions and the best possible care, an individual will commit suicide. The role of the care provider does not end there. Don't forget that suicide does not occur in a vacuum. Once the individual ends his or her life, there are clinicians, family members, friends and communities that may require support.

Death of a close friend or loved one is one of the most distressing and painful experiences of grief a person will face. Loss of someone to suicide can be especially devastating. Survivors often feel alone, isolated, overwhelmed and burdened with unanswerable questions concerning the person's death.

The expression and inner experience of grief is unique to each individual and is influenced by the person's past experiences, personality, family, culture, spiritual and religious beliefs, and traditional practices. Although there are no universally accepted rules governing what constitutes 'normal' grief, there are a number of recognized 'phases' that most people in mourning go through at some point in their grieving process:
- accepting that the loss is real
- allowing the pain of the loss to be experienced
- adjusting to a life without the deceased
- allowing oneself to resume living.

Experience of shock and disbelief is normal in the first few hours or days following the loss of a loved one. Once the initial shock of the

Suicide Risk Management: A Manual for Health Professionals, Second Edition.
Sonia Chehil and Stan Kutcher.
© 2012 John Wiley & Sons, Ltd. Published 2012 by John Wiley & Sons, Ltd.

loss has dissipated, most people slowly begin the process of recognizing and accepting the loss. Feelings of intense sadness, anger, hopelessness, helplessness and guilt often wax and wane throughout the day, with periods of extreme intensity becoming less overwhelming and less persistent over time. Thoughts about not wanting to be alive anymore, that life is not worth living, and of wanting to reunite with the deceased are not uncommon during this period.

After six months to one year, the pain associated with the grief generally becomes less intrusive, less intense and less persistent. Although there may be reexperiencing of intense grief when confronted with reminders of the loss, and periods of feeling sad, angry and empty, these grief experiences no longer prevent the person for moving on with their life and doing what they need to do, such as returning to work, returning to school, reconnecting in their personal relationships, participating in social and recreational activities, and caring for their families and children.

Grief for suicide survivors can be an intense and prolonged process. Grief may be complicated by feelings of intense guilt, anger, abandonment and shame. Survivors often struggle with trying to reconcile 'why' someone committed suicide – replaying the events leading to the death over and over, searching for clues to possible explanations. Many struggle with self-blame and are tormented by 'what if?' scenarios – searching for things they could have done differently or ruminating over things that were or were not said and things that were or were not done. Anger is also a common emotion experienced by survivors. Survivors may direct the anger at themselves, at the deceased or at others – particularly friends, care providers, teachers and family members who were in contact with the person before their death.

In addition, survivors are often burdened with having to deal with the social and cultural stigma of suicide. Stigma can intensify feelings of shame, humiliation and self-reproach for both individuals and families. Fear of social exclusion, ridicule, blame and judgment can lead survivors to silence themselves, hide the truth from others, withdraw from their social networks and avoid getting help and support. It can also lead close friends, family and other supports to distance themselves from the survivor.

Common feelings experienced by survivors
- despair
- sorrow
- shock
- disbelief
- abandonment
- guilt
- shame
- humiliation
- anger
- emotional numbness or detachment.
- loss of interest in daily activities or hobbies.

Most people think of grieving as being predominantly an emotional process but grieving also involves thinking and behavioural processes in the weeks to months following the death of a loved one.

Thinking or cognitive responses in grief include:
- flashbacks, nightmares and disturbing memories of the suicide
- difficulty concentrating and making decisions
- trouble accepting the reality of the suicide
- repeated visual images of one's loved one

Behavioral responses in grief include:
- difficulty coping at work, at home and in relationships
- trouble moving forward with one's life
- withdrawal from regular routines and activities, and social isolation
- avoidance of people who remind one of one's loved one
- sleep problems
- lack of motivation

People who have lost someone to suicide are at higher risk for depression and complicated grief, as well as for suicide. Most survivors slowly begin to feel better in the months following the loss of a loved one, and are eventually able to move forward with the support of friends and family. For some, the anguish and sorrow of grief does not abate with time and is so severe, so persistent and so long-lasting that they are unable to resume their lives – these individuals may be suffering from complicated grief, which requires professional assessment and treatment.

In complicated grief, the intensity, quality, pervasiveness and duration of the signs and symptoms of grieving are beyond what would be considered reasonable or expected given the individual's family, culture or social context. Complicated grief is associated with greater risk of clinical depression, anxiety disorder, substance abuse, poor general health and persistent psychosocial disability. Although grief shares many of the features of clinical depression – sadness, sleep problems, weight loss, loss of interest in things, social withdrawal, irritability, difficulties with focus and concentration – the symptoms of grief are less persistent, pervasive and impairing than those of clinical depression.

Suspect complicated grief if:

- grief symptoms last longer than expected and significantly interfere with the person's functioning
- grief symptoms are more severe and intense than expected and significantly interfere with the person's functioning
- symptoms develop that are not part of normal grief symptoms:
  o persistent thoughts of suicide
  o prolonged intense feelings of hopelessness
  o prolonged intense feelings of worthlessness
  o psychotic symptoms
  o new-onset or worsening problematic alcohol or drug use.

What can be done?

In many cases the person who has died by suicide leaves behind a family or significant other. In such cases it is important to offer support and counselling to these individuals. Many may feel guilty or personally responsible. Some may be angry at the person who suicided. Whatever the affect or thoughts, grief is an ongoing process with no definitive end. Although an individual may experience the loss differently as time goes on, bereaved individuals often report that the grieving process is never truly 'over'.

Severe grief can disrupt work, school and relationships, and impair a person's ability to care for children, complete household tasks and meet responsibilities and expectations. This is NORMAL. Most people are able to mobilize internal and external support systems and work through their loss without any outside intervention. Some people, particularly those without a strong support network, will benefit from supportive interventions or counselling to help them through their process of healing. Others may experience temporary emotional or physical symptoms that are particularly distressing, which may be amenable to treatment, such as sleep difficulties or severe anxiety. In such cases short-term use of a mild sedative may provide much-needed relief and facilitate the individual's ability to function. Medication, however, is not used as a treatment for grief.

Offering a short period of supportive counselling (one or two meetings) in which individuals are able to discuss the event and mourn their loss is useful. Often the most meaningful way to help someone who has experienced loss is to simply listen to them. Telling the story is one of the oldest healing arts. Bereaved individuals often feel compelled to tell and retell the story surrounding their loved one's life and death. Each time the story is repeated, the reality of the loss becomes increasingly undeniable. Telling and retelling moves the experience from the context of present tense into the context of the past and can aid in acceptance and moving forward.

These sessions can also help individuals to focus on practical issues that arise as a consequence of the suicide. For example, if a young child has been left by the suicide of a mother, what plans are being put into place for their proper care? Surviving children may need particular attention, and it is not unusual for them to experience a number of distressing symptoms, such as bad dreams, sleep difficulties, somatic distress and so on. For some children, a longer period of support and counselling may be needed. These services can be provided by mental health professionals but they may also be provided or augmented by religious or community organisations. If this is case, the mental health staff should communicate with those providing support and offer assistance in the form of training in useful therapeutic strategies if need be.

Some survivors may find interventions such as group support useful. In many communities, bereavement groups that are not specific for suicide can provide the support needed. Some communities have unique groups or organizations that are specific to those who have lost a family member or friend through suicide. Health providers should be aware of such community resources and be prepared to direct those who are interested in such support to the most appropriate resource available.

Remember: people who have lost someone to suicide are at higher risk for suicide, clinical depression and complicated grief.

Although the vast majority of people will journey through the grieving process successfully, some individuals may experience a complicated grief reaction and be at risk for clinical depression, anxiety, alcohol and substance abuse, and suicide. These individuals require an urgent comprehensive assessment and appropriate intervention.

Assessment of the suicide survivor:

- Make sure they feel safe and comfortable.
- Acknowledge and validate their feelings.
- Do not tell them not to cry or get angry.
- Do not tell them how you think they should feel.
- Give them space and time to talk about their loss.
- Gain an understanding of their past experiences with and reactions to loss.
- Gain an understanding of their family, culture, spiritual and religious beliefs, and expectations of the grieving process.
- Gain an understanding of the circumstances of their loss.
- Gain an understanding of the meaning and significance of the loss to the survivor.
- Gain an understanding of the support networks available to the survivor.
- ALWAYS look for symptoms that are not part of normal grieving.
- ALWAYS assess for suicide risk.
- ALWAYS look for signs of clinical depression and anxiety.
- ALWAYS look for signs of alcohol and drug abuse.

Management of the suicide survivor:

- Provide support and reassurance.
- Reinforce that the suicide was not their fault.
- Provide education about the grieving process.
- Assist problem-solving around practical issues and concerns.
- Encourage them to express how they feel but do not push them to talk about their experience or feelings if they are not ready.
- Encourage the remembering of positive experiences.
- Encourage them to connect with their social supports.
- Encourage their sharing with others who knew the deceased.

- Encourage normal routines and activities.
- Encourage self-care.
- Encourage realistic goal-setting.
- Consider the use of a mild sedative to assist with significant sleep difficulty or severe anxiety but do not use antianxiety or anti-depressant medications as a treatment for grief or as a substitute for verbal comfort and reassurance.
- Offer referral to available support services as appropriate.
- Continue to look for symptoms that are not part of normal grieving.
- ALWAYS assess for suicide risk.
- ALWAYS look for signs of clinical depression and anxiety.
- ALWAYS look for signs of alcohol and drug abuse.
- Provide short, frequent check-ins rather than longer, less-frequent visits as needed.
- Prepare them for times, such as anniversaries, religious festivals and celebrations, that are likely to evoke emotional reactions.

Chapter 9

Care for the Carer: Death of a Patient by Suicide

Sometimes, despite our best interventions and the best possible care, an individual will commit suicide.

The suicide of a patient can have a substantial impact on the health provider(s) responsible for the patient's care. Due to the nature of their work, health providers (particularly those who work in specialty mental health services) are at increased risk of being affected by the suicide of a patient. In some cases, the emotional reaction to the suicide of a patient can be profound and even professionally disabling. Clinicians who were close to the deceased are 'survivors' of suicide and can experience grief due to the loss just like any other survivor who was close to the deceased. In addition, clinicians are not immune to experiencing complicated grief, depression and suicidality in the wake of a suicide death.

Health-provider reactions to the suicide death of a patient may include

- shock
- guilt
- anger
- self-doubt
- self-reproach
- loss of confidence as a health provider
- feelings of incompetence
- fear of working with patients who may be suicidal

Suicide Risk Management: A Manual for Health Professionals, Second Edition.
Sonia Chehil and Stan Kutcher.
© 2012 John Wiley & Sons, Ltd. Published 2012 by John Wiley & Sons, Ltd.

- fear of being judged by or losing the respect of colleagues
- fear of being blamed by and losing the respect of the deceased family members.

Although it is not possible to mitigate all risk to health providers when they are faced with the suicide of a patient, there are a number of ways health providers can prepare themselves for the possible death of a patient by suicide and there are a number of approaches that can be taken by health care teams and health institutions to support clinicians who have been affected by the suicide death of a patient.

How to prepare yourself for working with suicidal patients

1 Be aware of your own thoughts and feelings about suicide and suicidal patients.

2 Acccpt that suicide is not always preventable.

3 Develop healthy strategies to effectively manage harmful emotional, psychological and behavioural reactions to the suicidal patient.

4 Be prepared emotionally, psychologically, personally and professionally for the death of a patient by suicide.

5 Talk to colleagues who work with high-risk patients about how they cope with and manage working with suicidal patients and how they have coped with and managed the death of a patient by suicide.

6 Be aware of the supports available to you if and when you need them.

7 Be confident in your ability to assess and manage suicide risk:
- know the 'warning signs' of acute suicide risk
- know the suicide risk and protective factors
- know the unique risk factors relevant to the populations you serve
- know how to ask patients about suicidality
- know how to determine suicide risk
- know how to manage suicide risk
- consult with peers for support, to debrief, for case reviews and to discuss clinical decision-making and case management
- know the services and supports available for patients in your jurisdiction and how these supports and services can be accessed
- know the laws governing consent, confidentiality, release of information and involuntary hospital admission in your jurisdiction.

What to do if your patient dies by suicide

1 Take care of your emotional, psychological, physical and personal needs.
2 Be aware of your thoughts, feelings and reactions to the death.
3 Remember that grief is a process and is unique to each individual.
4 Connect with your personal and professional network of supports.
5 Share and explore your thoughts and feelings with trusted colleagues.
6 Consult with peers for support, to debrief or to review the case.
7 Do not accept blame or blame yourself or others for the person's death.
8 Contact the family and loved ones and offer condolences.
9 Do not breach confidentiality.
10 Provide the family and loved ones with support if appropriate, or offer information and referral to other supports as needed.

Health care teams, colleagues and health institutions: what can you do?

Three principles of post-suicide interventions for health providers

1 support
2 learn
3 educate.

Support

Provide peer supports to health providers who have experienced the death of a patient by suicide. While this can often occur informally, health institutions and other health organizations should facilitate and encourage this support. Such support need not be overbearing; a quiet recognition of the situation and availability to discuss how they are feeling is usually all that is required. Administrators or senior clinicians must make a concerted effort to provide this support to any health care worker who reports to them. Often clinicians may blame themselves for the event or be shocked by it. Some people may respond by wanting to stop seeing patients. Others may become despondent. Gentle support will be much appreciated and very helpful.

Colleagues can help by:
- Being available to provide support.
- Encouraging sharing of thoughts and feelings when the person is ready.
- Providing perspective and normalizing the person's emotional, psychological and behavioural response.
- Being aware of the signs of complicated grief, depression and suicide.
- Supporting the person to regain professional confidence.

Some health providers may require additional support and intervention for emotional difficulties following the death of a patient by suicide. Ideally, this should be made available through ongoing health-assistance programs. If these are not available it should be the responsibility of the administration or senior clinicians to ensure that such support is available if needed.

Learn

It is always important to learn from the death of any patient, whatever the cause. Many hospitals have 'mortality rounds' in which objective review of fatal cases occurs as a learning exercise. In the case of suicide, case reviews should be conducted in a supportive and nonjudgemental manner and should follow prescribed procedures. Institutions and other health care organizations should have written policies, plans and procedures that address the above issues and should promote staff awareness of them. Such sessions should involve groups of clinicians and be chaired by a senior clinician. Recommendations arising from such reviews should be taken into consideration for policy or service directions.

Institutional mortality reviews should be cognizant of the emotional impact that a patient's suicide can have on a staff member and should ensure that these reviews are conducted in a respectful and confidential manner.

Educate

Promote training in suicide risk assessment and suicide interventions for all health providers, both during their professional training and as continuing health education courses. Health providers need to have competencies in suicide risk assessment. In addition to enhancing suicide risk assessment and care competencies, it is important that providers understand that even with the best clinical care, some patients will die by suicide.

All health providers should also receive education regarding: the laws governing consent, confidentiality, release of information and involuntary hospital admission in their jurisdiction; how to communicate effectively with the media; and how to support bereaved family members and loved ones, as well as colleagues.

Chapter 10
Clinical Vignettes for Group or Individual Study

Cases: suicide assessment

The cases in this chapter have been developed to provide the reader with an opportunity to practice their suicide-risk-assessment skills. They can be used for individual self-study or in a group-learning format.

For each case, apply the Tool for Assessment of Suicide Risk (TASR) and come to a conclusion as to the level of risk: high, moderate or low. Then address these issues:

- What can you decide now and what else do you need to know to inform further management?
- What will you do in this case? How are you going to manage the patient?
- How did the case affect you? How can you best address its impact on you?

If these cases are being used in a group format, the group should identify a facilitator. If an expert is available to the group then the expert could be used as either a facilitator or a resource person.

Case one

Mrs J.S. is a 35-year-old housewife with a 19-year history of depression. This is her third episode. In previous episodes she improved with

Suicide Risk Management: A Manual for Health Professionals, Second Edition.
Sonia Chehil and Stan Kutcher.
© 2012 John Wiley & Sons, Ltd. Published 2012 by John Wiley & Sons, Ltd.

antidepressant medications, usually within four to six weeks after beginning treatment. She has had no previous suicide attempts but her mother died of suicide many years ago. She is currently in a major depressive episode of some two months' duration and feels hopeless and worthless. She does not see any future for her children or herself and thinks that she would be better off dead. She is divorced and lives alone with her two sons, who are aged 8 and 6 years. She has been taking an antidepressant medication for about two weeks and her mood is subjectively no better but she has more energy. Her major complaint (the reason why she came to see you) is painful headaches and she wants 'lots of strong painkillers'. At her last visit a week ago she told you she 'did not want to live with the black dog of depression anymore'. Today she admits to feeling that 'life often does not seem worth living' and tells you that she has thoughts about killing herself. When you directly question her about suicidal plans she is vague and evasive in her response. When you ask how her children are doing she tells you that she has sent them to visit her ex-husband.

Case two

Mr M.I. is a 48-year-old unemployed male. About five weeks ago he had a heart attack from which he seems to have made a good recovery. He was discharged from the hospital about three weeks ago and has been at home since, mostly watching television and reading. He has come to see you complaining about back pain and constipation. At times during your interview he seems on the point of crying and he has told you that he is very unhappy with how things are turning out for him. He says that his friends tell him it is common to be depressed after a heart attack. He tells you that his biggest interest right now is the Church, in which he has been a member for over 20 years, and talks about how his faith is very important to him and is sustaining him at this point in his life. He tells you that he is worried that he is losing his faith and talks about frequent anxiety attacks. On direct questioning he admits to having frequent thoughts about killing himself by taking all his heart pills at once but is worried that he will go to hell if he does. Yesterday he took a gun from its drawer and sat looking at it for about 15 minutes trying to decide if he should kill himself. He decided that his faith would not let him do it and that his wife would suffer if he committed suicide so he put the gun away.

Case three

Mr T. is a 46-year-old unemployed male with a known history of alcohol abuse and depression. He had his last depressive episode about two years ago and he was lost to follow-up after successful treatment with an antidepressant. He has not seen any health professional for at least one year and presents today to the emergency room complaining of abdominal pain. A physical examination is unremarkable and an X-ray of the abdomen shows no pathological findings. He lives alone and denies using any alcohol or drugs in the last month. His main concerns are about his physical health and he presents a variety of vague complaints about headaches and back pain after he is told that there is nothing to find regarding his abdominal pain. He denies being depressed but becomes tearful when talking about going back to the street where he has been living. He asks for food and the emergency-room nurse complains that he is abusing the system.

Case four

Mrs C. is a 23-year-old single actress who has not been able to obtain steady work in her profession since she moved to this city some six months ago. She supports herself by waiting on tables in a local bar. She has cut her wrists with a kitchen knife after an argument with the bartender with whom she has been living for the last two weeks. This is the third episode of wrist-cutting she has experienced in the last three months. She also has cigarette burn marks on her upper arms and back and her face shows old bruises where she fell and hit her head while working. She does not have a history of depression or any other psychiatric disorder and before the abovementioned episodes no history of self-harm behaviours. She does not drink or use drugs and is uncomfortable at her apartment because her boyfriend 'drinks too much' and 'gets loud'. She complains about feeling sad but denies being hopeless. She says she did not want to kill herself but cut herself because she did not know what else she should do.

Case five

Mr M. is a 19-year-old male who has taken a handful of aspirin tablets after an argument with his mother. This is his fifth episode of self-harm (always taking 'pills') in three years. He has never had a psychiatric diagnosis and in all previous cases he refused to see a psychiatrist or failed to show up for appointments after being seen in the emergency room. He has been in trouble with the law for selling drugs and for stealing from stores. His mother is a well-known political figure and she tells you that he is always trying to manipulate her into doing what he wants and always trying to 'get attention'. He denies any depressive symptoms but demands that you tell his mother to let him transfer to a new school because at his current school 'all the teachers are assholes'.

He threatens to take more pills when he gets home if he is denied his demand.

Case six

Mrs P. is a 68-year-old woman with a five-year history of treated breast cancer. She lives with her 70-year-old husband, who is very supportive of her. Her eldest daughter, her son-in-law and her two grandchildren live next door. She is very close to them all and visits daily. She has just been diagnosed with a recurrence of her cancer and broke down in her doctor's office, crying and saying that she does not want to live anymore. She had a brief period of 'the blues' after her third child was born but has never been treated for any psychiatric problem. There is a strong history of depression in her biological family but no history of suicide. She denies having any suicidal plans and tells you that her thoughts about not wanting to live are gone. Now she feels embarrassed about having them and feels very upset. She denies feeling hopeless and wants to go home.

Case seven

Mr J. is a 34-year-old male who telephones the clinic and says (with slurred speech) that he is suicidal. He states that he has a gun and has decided to kill himself after he kills his wife and six-month-old child because 'they are possessed by the devil'. He wants the clinic doctor to come to the house and make sure that everyone is dead because that is the only way that he can think of to 'save their souls'.

Case eight

Mr R.J. is a 67-year-old bank executive and high-profile community leader. He is active in a number of health charities and is the financial controller at his church. He is well known to the hospital staff as he recently stepped down as chairman of the hospital board. This evening he presents to the emergency room with rapid onset of chest pain accompanied by respiratory distress, palpitations and thoughts that he will die. This episode came on suddenly as he and his wife were getting ready to go out to a cancer society fundraising dinner. It had largely resolved by the time he was assessed in the emergency room.

All investigations including EKG and cardiac enzymes are unremarkable. His wife, who had accompanied him to the hospital, has just left to 'go home and change clothes'. He asks to see you in private and confides that earlier that day he was informed by a physician in a confidential walk-in clinic in a distant location in the city that he was HIV positive, the result of an eight-month secret relationship with one of the teenage girls (a known sex worker and intravenous drug abuser) whom he had been 'counselling' through a church-based programme for street youth. He has not told anyone about what has happened and a counsellor at the walk-in clinic has asked him to come to an appointment tomorrow to discuss what he needs to do.

Mr R.J. has no personal or family history of mental illness and has never considered nor attempted suicide. He has had no significant medical illnesses and is taking no medications. However, since he received the news about his health status earlier today he has been having severe anxiety, numerous physical symptoms and is experiencing frequent suicidal thoughts that are intense but of short duration. He does not know what he should do. He is mortified at what this situation may do to his reputation and is convinced that he will be fired from his work. He feels guilty about his actions and does not know what he will tell his wife. He denies having a suicidal plan and does not want to keep his appointment at the clinic tomorrow, but instead thinks that he should 'go for a holiday to try and sort this out'.

Appendix A

Tool for Assessment of Suicide Risk (TASR)

Suicide Risk Management: A Manual for Health Professionals, Second Edition.
Sonia Chehil and Stan Kutcher.
© 2012 John Wiley & Sons, Ltd. Published 2012 by John Wiley & Sons, Ltd.

TOOL FOR ASSESSMENT OF SUICIDE RISK (TASR)

NAME: _____ Collateral: _____ Chart #: _____

INDIVIDUAL RISK PROFILE:	YES	NO
Demographics: Age/gender (in most jurisdictions: >65/15–35 yrs; M > F); culture; socioeconomic status	☐	☐
Family History: Suicide, suicide behaviours, psychiatric disorder	☐	☐
Past/Present Psychiatric Diagnosis: Mood, anxiety, psychotic, alcohol/drug, personality disorders	☐	☐
Medical Illness: Chronic, disabling, stigmatizing	☐	☐
Poor Social Supports: Living alone, isolated, poor social network, unhealthy relationships	☐	☐
Domestic Problems: Violence/abuse, relationship breakdown, conflict, pressure, dysfunction	☐	☐
Poor Stress Tolerance: Poor self-management, coping, problem-solving, decision-making skills	☐	☐
Past Suicide Behaviours: Suicide attempts, aborted attempts, self-harm	☐	☐
Past/Present Abuse: Recent or current abuse/violence; history of childhood abuse	☐	☐
Exposure to Suicide: Direct/indirect – peers, family, community, culture, social media	☐	☐

SYMPTOM RISK PROFILE:	YES	NO
Depression/Dysphoria	☐	☐
Hopelessness	☐	☐
Severe Anhedonia	☐	☐
Intense Emotion: Anxiety/panic, shame, humiliation, guilt, anger, isolation/loneliness	☐	☐
Shut Down: Emotional withdrawal, disengaged, noncommunicative	☐	☐
Severe Self-reproach/Worthlessness	☐	☐
Impaired Reasoning: Rigid thinking; poor judgement/problem-solving/decision-making	☐	☐
Poor Self-Control: Impulsivity; poor regulation of emotions and behaviours; violence/aggression	☐	☐
Psychosis: *Command hallucinations	☐	☐
Problematic Alcohol/Drug Use	☐	☐

INTERVIEW RISK PROFILE:	YES	NO
Suicide Ideation: Frequency, intensity, duration, persistence	☐	☐
Suicide Intent: Degree of ambivalence and expectation/commitment to die	☐	☐
Suicide Plan: Method, lethality, preparation	☐	☐
Concealed Suicidality: Warning signs, verbal/nonverbal cues, collateral, 'clinical intuition'	☐	☐
Past Suicide Attempt: Number, trigger, context, method, lethality, consequences	☐	☐
Access to Lethal Means: Availability of and accessibility to popular lethal methods	☐	☐
Recent Alcohol/Drug Consumption or Intoxication	☐	☐
Suicide Trigger: Recent, evolving or anticipated crisis/conflict/loss; victimization; trauma	☐	☐
Unsolvable Problem: Can't see any solution/unable or unwilling to search for alternatives	☐	☐
Intolerable State: Unbearable emotional/psychological/physical state or circumstance	☐	☐

RISK BUFFERS:		
Reasons for Living	☐	☐
Internal Strengths for Managing Risk	☐	☐
External Strengths for Managing Risk	☐	☐

LEVEL OF IMMEDIATE SUICIDE RISK: ☐ HIGH ☐ MODERATE ☐ LOW

Assessment Completed by: _____   DATE: _____

© Chehil & Kutcher, 2011

Appendix B

6-ITEM Kutcher Adolescent Depression Scale: KADS

6-ITEM
Kutcher Adolescent Depression Scale: KADS

NAME: _____   DATE: _____

OVER THE LAST WEEK, HOW HAVE YOU BEEN "ON AVERAGE" OR "USUALLY" REGARDING THE FOLLOWING ITEMS:

1. Low mood, sadness, feeling blah or down, depressed, just can't be bothered.

☐	☐	☐	☐
Hardly Ever	Much of The Time	Most of The Time	All of The Time

2. Feelings of worthlessness, hopelessness, letting people down, not being a good person.

☐	☐	☐	☐
Hardly Ever	Much of The Time	Most of The Time	All of The Time

3. Feeling tired, feeling fatigued, low in energy, hard to get motivated, have to push to get things done, want to rest or lie down a lot.

☐	☐	☐	☐
Hardly Ever	Much of The Time	Most of The Time	All of The Time

4. Feeling that life is not very much fun, not feeling good when usually (before getting sick) would feel good, not getting as much pleasure from fun things as usual (before getting sick).

☐	☐	☐	☐
Hardly Ever	Much of The Time	Most of The Time	All of The Time

5. Feeling worried, nervous, panicky, tense, keyed up, anxious.

☐	☐	☐	☐
Hardly Ever	Much of The Time	Most of The Time	All of The Time

6. Thoughts, plans or actions about suicide or self-harm.

☐	☐	☐	☐
Hardly Ever	Much of The Time	Most of The Time	All of The Time

1

© Dr Stan Kutcher, 2006

Suicide Risk Management: A Manual for Health Professionals, Second Edition.
Sonia Chehil and Stan Kutcher.
© 2012 John Wiley & Sons, Ltd. Published 2012 by John Wiley & Sons, Ltd.

6 - item KADS scoring:

In every item, score:

      a)   = 0
      b)   = 1
      c)   = 2
      d)   = 3

then add all 6 item scores to form a single Total Score.

Interpretation of total scores:

Total scores at or above 6 suggest 'possible depression' (and a need for more thorough assessment). Total scores below 6 indicate 'probable not depressed'.

Reference

- LeBlanc JC, Almudevar A, Brooks SJ, Kutcher S: Screening for Adolescent Depression: Comparison of the Kutcher Adolescent Depression Scale with the Beck Depression Inventory, Journal of Child and Adolescent Psychopharmacology, 2002 Summer; 12(2):113-26.

Self-report instruments commonly used to assess depression in adolescents have limited or unknown reliability and validity in this age group. We describe a new self-report scale, the Kutcher Adolescent Depression Scale (KADS), designed specifically to diagnose and assess the severity of adolescent depression. This report compares the diagnostic validity of the full 16-item instrument, brief versions of it, and the Beck Depression Inventory (BDI) against the criteria for major depressive episode (MDE) from the Mini International Neuropsychiatric Interview (MINI). Some 309 of 1,712 grade 7 to grade 12 students who completed the BDI had scores that exceeded 15. All were invited for further assessment, of whom 161 agreed to assessment by the KADS, the BDI again, and a MINI diagnostic interview for MDE. Receiver operating characteristic (ROC) curve analysis was used to determine which KADS items best identified subjects experiencing an MDE. *Further ROC curve analyses established that the overall diagnostic ability of a six-item subscale of the KADS was at least as good as that of the BDI and was better than that of the full-length KADS. Used with a cutoff score of 6, the six-item KADS achieved sensitivity and specificity rates of 92% and 71%, respectively—a combination not achieved by other self-report instruments. The six-item KADS may prove to be an efficient and effective means of ruling out MDE in adolescents.*

2

Appendix C
My Safety Plan

Suicide Risk Management: A Manual for Health Professionals, Second Edition.
Sonia Chehil and Stan Kutcher.
© 2012 John Wiley & Sons, Ltd. Published 2012 by John Wiley & Sons, Ltd.

MY SAFETY PLAN

If I have thoughts of harming myself or I am feeling hopeless or desperate I will start at STEP 1 and go through each step of my safety plan. Having this safety plan will help me focus on getting through this difficult time.

STEP 1: I will remind myself that:

- I am not alone – many people have thoughts of suicide.
- Thinking about suicide does not mean that I will do anything to harm myself.
- Thinking about suicide does not mean that I am weak.
- Thinking about suicide does not mean that I will lose control.
- I have strategies to get me through this.
- This feeling will not last forever.

STEP 2: I will use the following self-care strategies to comfort myself:

STEP 3: I will remind myself of my reasons for living:

STEP 4: I will tell someone, seek out support or call for help.

Friends/Family:

I will call/tell: PHONE#

If they are not available I will call/tell: PHONE#

If they are not available I will call/tell: PHONE#

Other Helper/Care Provider:

I will call: PHONE#

If they are not available I will call: PHONE#

STEP 5: I will get rid of anything I could use to hurt myself – pills, weapons, drugs, sharps...

STEP 6: I will not drink alcohol or use drugs.

STEP 7: I will make sure that I am somewhere safe.

1. I will go:

2. If I can't go there I will go:

3. If I can't go there I will go to the nearest Emergency Department

STEP 8: If I can't get somewhere safe I will call EMERGENCY SERVICES

Index

Suicide Risk Management: A Manual for Health Professionals, Second Edition.
Sonia Chehil and Stan Kutcher.
© 2012 John Wiley & Sons, Ltd. Published 2012 by John Wiley & Sons, Ltd.

Index compiled by Terry Halliday

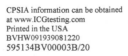